M000220872

UNIPAC Three: *Assessment and Treatment of Pain in the Terminally Ill*

Second Edition

Porter Storey, MD, FACP, FAAHPM
Associate Professor of Medicine
Section of Geriatrics
Baylor College of Medicine

Consultant in the Department of Symptom Control and Palliative Care
University of Texas MD Anderson Cancer Center

Medical Director
Palliative Care Services
St. Luke's Episcopal Hospital
Houston, Texas

Carol F. Knight, EdM
Knight Consultants
Austin, Texas

AAHPM

American Academy of Hospice and Palliative Medicine

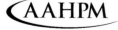

Mary Ann Liebert, Inc. publishers

The information presented and opinions expressed herein are those of the authors and do not necessarily represent the views of the sponsor or its parent agencies, the National Institutes of Health, the United States Public Health Service, the reviewers, or a consensus of the members of the American Academy of Hospice and Palliative Medicine. Any recommendations made by the authors must be weighed against the physician's own clinical judgment, based on but not limited to such factors as the patient's condition, benefits versus risks of suggested treatment, and comparison with recommendations of pharmaceutical compendia and other authorities.

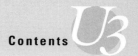

Contents

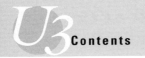

Contents

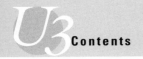
Contents

Tables

Figures

Acknowledgments

The authors and the American Academy of Hospice and Palliative Medicine (AAHPM) are deeply grateful to the following reviewers for their participation in the development of this component of the Academy's self-study curriculum, *Hospice/Palliative Care Training for Physicians: UNIPACs.* The reviewers' extensive comments and thoughtful suggestions greatly improved its contents. We want to express special gratitude to Doctors Smith, Finn, Holman, and Perencevich for coordinating local field testing of the first edition of the UNIPAC. And, finally, we wish to express special thanks to all of the practicing physicians, fellows, residents, and medical students who participated in the development and evaluation of this component of the Academy's physician training programs.

John W. Finn, MD
Past President
Board of Directors, AAHPM
Medical Director
Hospice of Michigan
Southfield, Michigan

Gerald H. Holman, MD
Founding Chairman
Board of Trustees, AAHPM
Amarillo, Texas

Eli N. Perencevich, DO
Clinical Assistant
Professor of Medicine
Ohio State University
Former Medical Director
Hospice of Columbus
Columbus, Ohio

Julia L. Smith, MD
Division Chief, Oncology/Hematology
Genessee Hospital
Associate Professor
Oncology in Medicine
University of Rochester Cancer Center
Medical Director
Hospice of Rochester
Rochester, New York

Academy's Physician Training Programs

The Academy recognizes the need for physician education on palliative medicine at the end of life and has designed its physician training programs to meet its own education goals, as well as those of the National Cancer Institute. The training programs include the following:

Hospice/Palliative Medicine: Self-Study Program for Physicians

The Academy's self-study program consists of a series of monographs, or UNIPACs, each of which follows the recommended format for self-instructional learning, including behavioral objectives, a pretest, reading material, clinical situations for demonstrating knowledge application, a posttest, and references. The self-study program was made possible with federal funds from the National Cancer Institute's Cancer Education Grant Program, Grant CA66771. The following UNIPACs are approved for CME credit:

- *UNIPAC One: The Hospice/Palliative Medicine Approach to End-of-Life Care*

- *UNIPAC Two: Alleviating Psychological and Spiritual Pain in the Terminally Ill*

- *UNIPAC Three: Assessment and Treatment of Pain in the Terminally Ill*

- *UNIPAC Four: Management of Selected Non-pain Symptoms in the Terminally Ill*

- *UNIPAC Five: Caring for the Terminally Ill—Communication and the Physician's Role on the Interdisciplinary Team*

- *UNIPAC Six: Ethical and Legal Decision Making When Caring for the Terminally Ill*

- *UNIPAC Seven: The Hospice/Palliative Medicine Approach to Caring for Patients with AIDS*

- *UNIPAC Eight: The Hospice/Palliative Medicine Approach to Caring for Pediatric Patients*

Although the UNIPACs may be used when studying for the American Board of Hospice and Palliative Medicine's written examination for certification, they were not developed for that purpose. The Academy recommends that candidates for the examination review selected references listed at the end of each UNIPAC and other materials relevant to the examination.

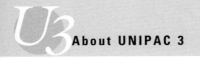

Pocket Guide to Hospice/Palliative Medicine

The *Pocket Guide to Hospice/Palliative Medicine* is a concise, clinically oriented reference for residents and practicing physicians. It consists primarily of tables and assessment tools from the Academy's self study program, *Hospice/Palliative Medicine: A Self-Study Program for Physicians.* Development of the Pocket Guide was made possible with federal funds from the National Cancer Institute's Cancer Education Grant Program, Grant CA66771.

Hospice and Palliative Medicine: Core Curriculum and Review Syllabus

The Academy's core curriculum and review syllabus, *Hospice and Palliative Medicine: Core Curriculum and Review Syllabus,* presents the core elements of hospice and palliative medicine identified by the Institute of Medicine as essential for effective end-of-life care. The document consists of a series of modules, each of which includes a brief narrative summary of a specific topic, objectives, and references. The curriculum was the first one in the United States developed primarily by palliative medicine physicians.

Primer of Palliative Care

The *Primer of Palliative Care* is a brief introduction to palliative care that covers the history of hospice, the basic elements of hospice and palliative care, pain and symptom management techniques, and alleviation of psychological, social, and spiritual distress. The Primer includes an annotated bibliography.

For more information on the Academy's physician training programs, call the AAHPM at (847) 375-4712 or fax (847) 375-6312.

Continuing Medical Education

Purpose

A UNIPAC is a packet of information formatted as a self-study program. It includes learning objectives, a pretest, reading material, clinical situations for demonstrating knowledge application, a posttest, and references. This self-study program is intended for physicians and physicians-in-training. It is designed to increase competence in palliative medical interventions for improving a patient's quality of life, particularly as death approaches. Specific, practical information is presented to help physicians assess and manage selected problems. After reading the UNIPAC, physicians are encouraged to seek additional training in hospice/palliative medicine.

Learning Objectives

Upon completion of this continuing medical education program, a physician should be better able to:

- Assess for the presence of cancer-related and noncancer-related pain.

- Identify social, emotional, and spiritual pain.

- Differentiate bone, neuropathic, and visceral pain.

- Prescribe appropriate adjuvant drugs to treat bone, neuropathic and visceral pain, and pain due to raised intracranial pressure.

- Calculate oral morphine equivalents of codeine, oxycodone, and hydromorphone.

- Calculate a continuous subcutaneous-infusion dose of morphine and hydromorphone.

- Calculate an appropriate starting dose of morphine therapy for an opioid-naive patient.

- Prescribe an appropriate alternative route of drug administration.

- Prescribe appropriate treatments for nausea and constipation associated with opioid use.

Recommended Procedure

To receive maximum benefit from this UNIPAC, the following procedure is recommended:

- Complete the pretest before reading the UNIPAC.

- Review the learning objectives.

- Study each section and the clinical situations.

- Review the correct responses to the pretest.

- Complete the posttest by marking your answers on the answer sheet.

Accreditation Statement

The American Academy of Hospice and Palliative Medicine (AAHPM) is accredited by the Accreditation Council for Continuing Medical Education (ACCME) to provide continuing medical education for physicians.

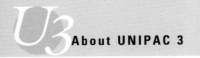

The AAHPM designates this continuing medical education activity for a maximum of six (6) hours in Category 1 towards the AMA Physician's Recognition Award.

Physicians are eligible to receive credit by completing and returning the evaluation form and the posttest answer sheet to the AAHPM. The Academy will keep a record of AMA/PRA Category 1 credit hours and the record will be provided on request; however, physicians are responsible for reporting their own Category 1 CME credits when applying for the AMA/PRA or for other certificates or credentials. Each physician should claim only those hours of credit that he or she actually spent in the activity.

Disclosure

All faculty are required to disclose to program participants any relationship, including financial interest or affiliation(s), with a commercial company, as well as discussion of unlabeled uses. The program authors have disclosed information on sources of funding for research, consulting agreements, offices in professional associations, financial interests, and stock ownership.

Porter Storey, MD, once served on the speakers' bureau for Purdue Pharmaceuticals and has received research support from the National Cancer Institute. **Carol F. Knight, EdM,** has received research support from the National Cancer Institute.

Review and Revision

Reviewed and re-approved by the American Academy of Hospice and Palliative Medicine's Publications and CME Committees: May 2002.

Term of Offering

The release date for the second edition of this UNIPAC is April, 2003, and the expiration date is December 31, 2006. Final date to request credit is December 31, 2006.

Posttest Pass Rate

The posttest pass rate is 75%.

Additional Information

Additional information is available from the American Academy of Hospice and Palliative Medicine, where staff can direct you to physicians specializing in end-of-life care.

This self-study program was supported in part by federal funds from the National Cancer Institute's Cancer Education Grant Program, Grant CA66771.

Evaluation Form

Use this evaluation form to rate the UNIPAC that you have completed according to the five criteria listed below and then mail or fax the form to the Academy at the address below. To receive CME credit, follow the same procedure.

Currency of information	__Excellent	__Good	__Fair	__Poor
Clarity of presentation	__Excellent	__Good	__Fair	__Poor
Content of material	__Excellent	__Good	__Fair	__Poor
Effectiveness of teaching method	__Excellent	__Good	__Fair	__Poor
Relevance to my practice	__Excellent	__Good	__Fair	__Poor

Suggestions for improving the enduring material:

Mail or fax to:
American Academy of Hospice and Palliative Medicine
4700 W. Lake Avenue
Glenview, Illinois 60025-1485
Fax: 847/375-4777

CAAHPM

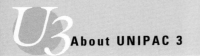
Pretest

Before proceeding, read each item and circle the one correct response.

1. **Pain described as "shooting" or "stabbing" often results from damage to:**

    A. Bones

    B. Nerves

    C. Brain

    D. Viscera

2. **The WHO ladder of oral opioids and adjuvants has been shown to provide relief in what percent of cancer patients:**

    A. 99%

    B. 90%

    C. 75%

    D. 50%

3. **In the palliative care setting, analgesics of choice include which of the following:**

    A. Hydromorphone

    B. Meperidine

    C. Pentazocine

    D. Propoxyphene

4. **Neuropathic cancer pain is usually responsive to which of the following:**

    A. Morphine alone

    B. NSAIDs

    C. NSAIDs and morphine

    D. Antidepressant and morphine

5. **Opioids prescribed for pain frequently cause clinically significant:**

    A. Addiction

    B. Respiratory depression

C. Itching

D. Constipation

6. **When patients are unable to swallow opioids, which of the following is an effective treatment:**

   A. Transdermal morphine

   B. Subcutaneous hydromorphone

   C. Nebulized methadone

   D. Rectal propoxyphene

7. **Patients treated with opioids should receive routine prophylaxis for which side effect:**

   A. Constipation

   B. Sedation

   C. Itching

   D. Myoclonus

8. **Anticholinergic drugs help with which of the following pain syndromes:**

   A. Bony

   B. Neuropathic

   C. Visceral

   D. Central

9. **In relation to oral morphine, injectable morphine is about:**

   A. Equally potent

   B. Ten times as potent

   C. Five times as potent

   D. Three times as potent

10. **Methadone should be used for relieving cancer pain when the patient has not obtained relief from:**

    A. Codeine or hydrocodone

    B. Very high dose IV/SC morphine

    C. Multidrug spinal infusions

    D. Rhizotomy or singulotomy

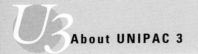

11. Patients often describe bone pain as:

    A. Shooting

    B. Deep and aching

    C. Spasms or cramping

    D. Colicky

12. Which of the following classes of drugs can be effective adjuvants to morphine when treating specific types of pain?

    A. NSAIDs

    B. Anticonvulsants

    C. Anticholinergics

    D. All the above

13. To calculate an effective initial daily dose of subcutaneous hydromorphone (Dilaudid), divide the patient's daily dose of oral morphine by:

    A. 20

    B. 3

    C. 5

    D. 2

14. When titrating morphine, the 24-hour dose can never be raised by more than:

    A. 10%

    B. 25%

    C. 50%

    D. None of the above

15. When bone pain occurs, which of the following may be an effective adjuvant to morphine?

    A. Ibuprofen

    B. Naproxen

    C. Valdecoxib (Bextra)

    D. All of the above

16. To calculate the equivalent parenteral dose of 30 mg of oral morphine, divide the oral dose of morphine by:

    A. 1.5

    B. 2.0

    C. 3

    D. 6

17. When titrating morphine, the most appropriate booster or increment dose for a patient receiving a baseline dose of 30 mg every 4 hours is:

    A. 2 to 5 mg

    B. 10 to 15 mg

    C. 20 to 39 mg

    D. None of the above

18. When pain related to nerve damage or dysesthesia occurs, which of the following may be an effective adjuvant to morphine:

    A. Nortriptyline (Pamelor, Aventyl)

    B. Scopolamine

    C. Ranitidine (Zantac)

    D. Naproxen

19. A patient is receiving 60 mg of oral morphine per day. The equivalent daily dose of parenteral hydromorphone (Dilaudid) is:

    A. 30 mg

    B. 20 mg

    C. 5 mg

    D. 3 mg

20. The use of morphine or other opioids appropriate for treating moderate to severe pain should be saved for the last few weeks or days of the patient's life due to the risk of:

    A. Addiction

    B. Tolerance

    C. Respiratory depression

    D. None of the above

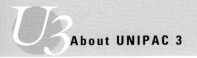

21. When the common side effect of constipation occurs as a result of opioid therapy, an appropriate first step is:

   A. Digital disimpaction

   B. Soap suds enema

   C. Trial of docusate

   D. Inquire about previous laxative use

22. Most terminally ill patients on opioid therapy require individually titrated doses of potent bowel stimulants such as:

   A. Senna

   B. Sorbitol

   C. Psyllium

   D. Docusate (Colace)

23. Types of pain that can contribute to a patient's experience of total pain include:

   A. Physical pain

   B. Social pain

   C. Spiritual pain

   D. All the above

24. When a home hospice patient can no longer swallow, which of the following is a preferred alternative route of opioid administration:

   A. Sublingual

   B. Intravenous

   C. Intramuscular

   D. Epidural

25. When treating pain caused by raised intracranial pressure, an effective adjuvant to morphine would be:

   A. Strontium 89

   B. Acetaminophen

   C. Dexamethasone

   D. Hydromorphone

26. Which of the following most commonly occurs with opioid therapy?

    A. Myclonus

    B. Delirium

    C. Urinary incontinence

    D. Drowsiness

27. An effective dose of immediate-release oral morphine provides pain relief for about:

    A. 2 hours

    B. 3 hours

    C. 4 hours

    D. 6 hours

28. Effective pain management is dependent on a comprehensive assessment of the causes of:

    A. Noncancer-related pain

    B. Cancer-related pain

    C. Nonphysical pain

    D. All of the above

29. One oxycodone 5 mg and acetaminophen 325 mg tablet is roughly equivalent to:

    A. 3 mg of oral morphine

    B. 7.5 mg oral morphine

    C. 15 mg oral morphine

    D. 4 mg oral hydromorphone

30. Visceral spasm pain can be effectively treated with:

    A. An opioid plus sorbital

    B. An opioid plus metoclopraminde

    C. An opioid plus oxybutynin

    D. Metoclopramide alone

Despite the publication of hundreds of articles on the assessment and treatment of pain, many dying patients continue to suffer from unrelieved pain during their last months of life. Of cancer patients with pain, 40% to 50% report moderate to severe pain, and 25% to 30% describe their pain as very severe.[1]

Most terminally ill patients experience several different types of pain. Twycross found that 80% of advanced cancer patients suffered from more than one type of pain, and 34% experienced four or more types of pain, each of which demanded a different set of treatments.[2] It has been estimated that at least 25% of all cancer patients die without adequate pain relief.[2]

Because most pain experienced during the terminal phases of life can be managed using relatively simple techniques, the question remains, why do so many patients continue to suffer? A study of pain in HIV disease illustrates this point: A group of AIDS patients was hospitalized with intractable pain and received daily physician visits, but their pain remained uncontrolled. A specialized pain team was asked to consult and, after assessing the patients, the team ordered oral morphine on a 24-hour around-the-clock schedule. The results of opioid therapy were described as dramatic, and most of the patients experienced relief from their pain.[3]

Prescribing oral morphine on a 24-hour around-the-clock schedule is one of the most basic techniques of pain control. Why are specialized pain teams often needed to initiate such fundamental techniques? Possible reasons include the following:

- Continued physician unfamiliarity with pain assessment and treatment

- Continued belief in misconceptions about morphine

- Undue concern about addiction issues, regulatory body reprimands, and lawsuits concerning the use of opioids

Three Basic Principles of Pain Assessment and Management

Cancer pain can be managed effectively in up to 90% of patients[1] by following the basic principles of effective pain management and by using relatively simple pain management techniques.

Effective pain management is a continuous three-step process, the first step being a thorough assessment of all types of pain that the patient is experiencing. The second step is treating each type of pain with individualized, type-specific interventions, and the third step involves continuous reassessment of the patient's pain and the efficacy of pre-

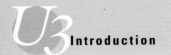
scribed treatments. When pain increases or remains uncontrolled, a thorough assessment is reinstituted and type-specific treatments are prescribed until all types of pain are adequately controlled.

The three basic principles of pain management are:

1. Assess for multiple causes of pain.

2. Treat each type of pain.

3. Reassess continuously, especially when pain remains uncontrolled.

Many dying patients experience *total pain*, a combination of four different types of pain, each of which interacts with the others and can result in all-encompassing pain or suffering. The four components of total pain, as described by Dr. Cicely Saunders, MD, are:

- Physical pains, usually multiple
- Emotional or psychic pain
- Social or interpersonal pain
- Spiritual or existential pain

When assessing for multiples causes of pain, the first step in the assessment process is to complete a careful history and physical, maneuvers that are most likely to reveal important information about the patient's pain without causing additional pain and expense.

An effective assessment employs careful listening, open-ended questioning, and the use of individualized patient-completed pain assessment scales to correctly identify each pain's location, intensity, and etiology.

Assess for Multiple Causes of Pain

A complete assessment is the essential first step in pain management—it is the building block upon which rests effective pain management. Assessments should include a history, physical, and the use of a numerical or visual analogue pain assessment scale, all tools that encourage patient communication about each pain's location, intensity, and etiology regardless of source. Laboratory, radiographic, and imaging studies may also be useful, but they are not substitutes for a thorough and compassionate assessment interview.

Assess for Pain from Three Sources

- Assess for pain caused by noncancer-related physical conditions.
- Assess for different specific types of cancer-related physical pain.
- Assess for nonphysical causes of pain.

Although a complete assessment may take an hour or two, it is time well spent. During the initial assessment process, correctly identifying the type and severity of pain from

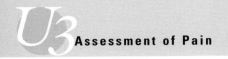
each source and measuring its severity result in more immediate provision of appropriate treatments and more rapid relief from pain. Hurried, incomplete assessments often fail to identify the presence of multiple causes of pain, such as neuropathic pain and spiritual pain, in which case the patient's unidentified spiritual agony may interfere with efforts to relieve the patient's equally severe neuropathic pain. During the assessment process, it is also important to determine the efficacy of current analgesic prescriptions.

Use Pain Assessment Scales

Although pain assessment scales can be time consuming to complete and in some cases may be viewed as an imposition by the patient, the use of patient-completed scales is invaluable, particularly when difficulties with verbal communication affect the patient's ability to adequately report pain and when concerns arise about the efficacy of ongoing pain control measures. The results obtained on numerical scales can be used in outcome studies to determine the effectiveness of various pain control measures.[4] See examples of pain assessment scales in the publications *Pocket Guide to Hospice and Palliative Medicine* and UNIPAC Eight.

The use of a specific type of scale is less important than ensuring that the scale is:

- Completed by the patient rather than by an observer
- Flexible enough to be adapted to the needs of a particular patient
- Simple enough to be used regularly
- Used consistently with the patient

Adapting the scale to each patient is vital. Children may respond to scales developed for children, such as the Bieri Faces Scale,[5] but patients from other cultures may find it easier to respond to individualized symbols for pain, for instance to a series of pictures of fires that are larger and larger. Regardless of which scale is used, it is important to continue using the same scale with the same patient to ensure reliability.

Remember Needs of Special Populations

Children, patients from other cultures, and patients with HIV disease are three population groups that require extra care during the assessment process.

Children and Patients from Other Cultures

Because children and non-English speaking patients from other cultures may have difficulty describing their pain verbally or rating it in terms of numerical pain assessment scales, extra care must be taken to ensure that their pain is adequately assessed.[6]

Children

When assessing pain in children, careful attention should be paid to the following issues:

- The child's developmental stage and its effect on the meanings of pain
- The child's developmental stage and its effect on the meaning of the child's prognosis
- The child–parent relationship
- The common occurrence of regression, i.e., increased dependency during profound illness

See *UNIPAC Eight: The Hospice/Palliative Medicine Approach to Caring for Pediatric Patients.*

Patients from Other Cultures

When assessing pain in patients from other cultures, careful attention should be paid to the following issues:

- Cultural differences in the meanings of pain
- Cultural differences in religious practices
- Cultural expectations regarding reactions to pain, i.e., stoicism or emotional expression

Patients with HIV Disease

Patients with HIV disease present special assessment challenges because, as a group, they experience unusual amounts of social, psychological, and spiritual pain resulting from conditions such as:

- Social isolation and blaming
- Chronic serial grief from the loss of many loved ones

See *UNIPAC Seven: The Hospice/Palliative Medicine Approach to Caring for Patients with HIV/AIDS.*

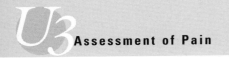

Listen Carefully During the Assessment Process

During the assessment process, careful and attentive listening can achieve the following:

- Encourage patients to provide information that helps identify multiple causes of pain
- Reassure both the patient and family of the physician's interest in the patient's total pain
- Demonstrate the physician's confidence that something can be done to control pain

Assess for Pain Caused by Noncancer-related Physical Conditions

During the assessment process, look for pain caused by preexisting and noncancer-related conditions, e.g., arthritis, bladder spasms, constipations, decubiti, migraine headaches, oral thrush, surgery, and injuries.

Assess for Specific Types of Cancer-related Physical Pain

An effective assessment depends on the physician's ability to differentiate cancer-related pains so that type-specific treatments can be initiated. Because patients frequently experience several different types of cancer-related pain concurrently, the adjectives that they use can help to identify each type of pain.

Bone Pain and Soft Tissue Pain

Bone pain intensifies on movement and is often tender to palpation. As with soft tissue pain, it is often described as "tender" or "deep and aching."

Neuropathic or Nerve Damage Pain

This type of pain is often described as "shooting," "burning," "stabbing, or "scalding." It usually follows the distribution of a sensory nerve and may present with allodynia (pain from light touch or mild pressure).

Raised Intracranial Pressure Pain

This type of pain is often described as generalized or posterior head pain and is usually accompanied by nausea.

Visceral Pain

These pains may be described as "spasms," "cramping," or "colicky."

Assess for Nonphysical Causes of Pain

Pain is not simply a matter of an impulse traveling along a nerve; it is much more. Total pain, a term used to describe the all-encompassing pain sometimes experienced by terminally ill patients, is a combination of four different types of pain (Table 1). Because each component of total pain interacts with the others, hospice/palliative medicine can be effective only if it addresses all four components.

Terminally ill patients frequently harbor death-related anxieties and fears, but may be reluctant to discuss them for fear their thoughts and feelings might be considered strange or abnormal. Physicians should inquire carefully about the presence of psychological,

---

Table 1: Four Components of Total Pain

P **Physical** problems, often multiple, must be specifically diagnosed and treated.[7]

A **Anxiety**, anger, and depression are critical components of pain that must be addressed by the physician in conjunction with other healthcare professionals.

I **Interpersonal problems**, including loneliness, financial stress, and family tensions, which are often interwoven in the fabric of a patient's symptoms.

N **Nonacceptance** of approaching death, a sense of hopelessness, and a desperate search for meaning can cause severe suffering that is unrelieved by medications.

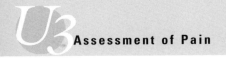

social, and spiritual pain and help normalize their presence by providing reassurance that most patients have similar concerns. With nonjudgmental listening and a caring presence, physicians can provide emotional support that sometimes is more important than additional tests or medications.

During the assessment process, estimating the severity of nonphysical pain is as important as rating the severity of cancer-related physical pain. Nonjudgmental listening and education often can alleviate mild nonphysical pain, but the presence of moderate to severe nonphysical pain calls for more potent interventions, such as the involvement of counselors, social workers, or chaplains, and the addition of pharmacological therapies when anxiety or depression interfere with quality of life.

Use Open-ended Assessment Questions

It is important to use open-ended questions to assess for the presence of nonphysical pain. Examples of open-ended questions that may elicit information about psychosocial and spiritual pain include the following:

- When people become seriously ill, they usually find themselves wondering why it happened to them. When you wonder about it, what comes to mind?

- When you think about the next few weeks or months, what are some of the concerns that come to your mind first? What things concern you more than others?

- When you think back over the years, what are some of your happiest times? Saddest?

- What has given you strength in the past? What gives you strength now? What do you wish could happen to give you more strength?

- How has this illness affected you emotionally? What has been particularly difficult? Has anything been more (less) difficult than you thought it might be?

- How is your family coping with this illness? Can you tell me something about what is going on with them? What are some of your concerns about your family?

Effective treatment of total pain depends on thorough assessments and specific interventions designed to relieve each type of pain. Most physical pain can be managed with relatively simple techniques, but effective control requires individualized treatment and medication dosages adequate to control the intensity of the pain being experienced.

In most cases, the practitioner can control pain adequately by:

- Following the World Health Organization's process for titrating oral pharmacological therapy
- Correctly calculating oral and injectable morphine equivalents
- Using effective starting doses and titrating upward as needed
- Using appropriate adjuvant drugs to treat each type of pain
- Anticipating problems with treatment, such as constipation or sedation
- Incorporating nonpharmacological methods, such as distraction and relaxation

Treating severe nonphysical pain and suffering presents a more challenging task for most physicians, but the following can be helpful:

- Involving all members of the interdisciplinary team, including the chaplain, social worker, and other counselors with expertise in grief-related issues
- Using pharmacological therapy to treat disabling anxiety and depression
- Offering supportive and caring presence while the patient searches for renewed hope, purpose, and meaning

Treat Pain Caused by Noncancer-related Physical Conditions

Because full descriptions of appropriate treatments for noncancer-related sources of pain can be found elsewhere, this UNIPAC offers only the following brief suggestions. (For more information on the treatment of constipation, see "Anticipate Problems with Opioid Treatment" on page 35.)

- **Arthritis:** Consider the use of nonsteroidal anti-inflammatory drugs (NSAIDs) or disease modifying agents
- **Bladder spasms:** Urinary retention may require a decrease in anticholinergic drugs or a Foley catheter. An irritated bladder may require antibiotics, pyridium, and/or oxybutynin (Ditropan) for relief.

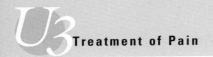

- **Constipation:** Consider the use of laxatives and other appropriate therapies. See "Anticipate Problems with Opioid Treatment," on page 35.

- **Decubiti:** Consider regular turning, special mattresses, and other appropriate treatments. If pain interferes with movement, prescribe analgesics prior to turning.

- **Migraine headaches:** Consider the use of antidepressants, ergot derivatives, selective serotonin agonists such as sumatriptan (Imitrex) and other appropriate therapies.

- **Muscle strain:** Consider massage, heating pads, relaxants, and other appropriate therapies.

- **Oral thrush:** Consider topical or systemic antifungals.

- **Surgery and injuries:** Consider physical therapy, opioids, and other appropriate analgesics.

Treat Specific Types of Cancer-related Physical Pain

Use Specific Interventions for Each Type of Cancer-related Physical Pain

Bone Pain and Soft Tissue Pain

Soft tissue pain usually responds well to opioid treatment. Bone pain is responsive to opioids but also may require an adjuvant drug. See "Use Adjuvant Drugs When Necessary" on page 40.

Neuropathic or Nerve Damage Pain

Adjuvant drugs are usually necessary because neuropathic pain often does not respond completely to opioids.

Raised Intracranial Pressure Pain

This type of pain may not respond completely to opioids and often requires the use of a steroid.

Visceral Pain or Colic Pain

These pains may respond completely to opioids, but adjuvant drugs, such as anticholinergics, can be very helpful in some cases.

Dispel Misconceptions about Opioids

Many physicians are reluctant to prescribe opioids due to misconceptions about their effects. Nurses may be reluctant to administer (and patients may be reluctant to use) morphine or other opioids for many of the same reasons. Correct responses to the most common misconceptions about morphine and other opioids include the following:[8]

Opioids ≠ Respiratory Depression

Clinically significant respiratory depression is extremely rare when patients receive optimal doses of an opioid. When opioids are carefully titrated, they are safe analgesics, even for patients with respiratory disease. Morphine has been shown to be safe and effective for treating the dyspnea associated with cancer[9,10] and chronic obstructive pulmonary disease.[11]

Due to concerns about respiratory depression, some physicians recommend the use of naloxone whenever respirations drop below 12 per minute; however, the use of naloxone is inappropriate in most of these cases. Many terminally ill patients experience respirations of 6 to 12 per minute when asleep or awake. Clinically significant respiratory depression may be suspected when both the patient's level of consciousness and respirations drop concomitantly, with respirations reaching <6 per minute; however, as long as the patient is arousable and/or breathing >6 per minute, naloxone should not be administered. Simple dosage reduction is usually adequate if the patient is truly overmedicated. See "Opioid Overdose" on page 40.

When terminally ill patients who have been on stable doses of opioids for several days develop the symptoms listed below, the normal dying process has begun. The appropriate action is to talk with the patient's family about the dying process, not to order naloxone.

Common symptoms of dying include decreased or erratic respirations, in conjunction with:

- Extreme weakness
- Decreased alertness, usually with confusion
- Cool extremities

(A few terminally ill patients die in a hyperventilatory state as a result of sepsis, acidosis, or respiratory muscle fatigue.)

Opioids ≠ Addiction

Physical dependence is an expected result of long-term opioid treatment, but it should not be confused with addiction.[1] Addiction is an extremely rare occurrence when opioids are administered to cancer patients in regularly scheduled and individually titrated doses.[12] When radiation or other treatments eliminate pain, opioids can be tapered off without withdrawal symptoms in the vast majority of patients. Many patients who fear addiction are reassured by the fact that opioid doses can be tapered off easily if their pain is relieved by treatments such as radiation.

Definitions:[13]

Addiction: Addiction is a primary, chronic, neurobiologic disease, with genetic, psychosocial, and environmental factors influencing its development and manifestations. It is characterized by behaviors that include one or more of the following: impaired control over drug use, compulsive use, continued use despite harm, and craving.

Physical dependence: Physical dependence is a state of adaptation that is manifested by a drug-class-specific withdrawal syndrome that can be produced by abrupt cessation, rapid dose reduction, decreasing blood level of the drug, and/or administration of an antagonist.

Opioids ≠ Rapid Tolerance

Tolerance is a state of adaptation in which exposure to a drug induces changes that result in a diminution of one or more of the drug's effects over time. Due to concerns about tolerance, many physicians save the use of opioids for the very end of a patient's life. However, the presence of unrelieved pain, not the patient's prognosis, should determine when opioids are used. Clinically significant tolerance is unusual because the therapeutic range of opioids is very wide. After an effective baseline dose is established, dose requirements usually plateau until disease progression occurs, at which time increased doses are necessary to control increased levels of pain.

Opioids ≠ Imminent Death

Many patients and family members are reluctant to use opioids because they equate their use with imminent death. By refusing opioids, patients and family members may think that they can magically forestall death. Due to their own concerns about tolerance and addiction, physicians may inadvertently reinforce this misconception and contribute to increased suffering by withholding opioids until the very end of a patient's life. Because pain is both psychologically and physically destructive, unrelieved pain may actually shorten survival time.

Opioids ≠ Narrow Effective Dose Range

Opioids have a very wide effective dose range. Two milligrams of oral morphine every 4 hours may be an effective dose for some patients, while others may require more than

300 mg every 4 hours. When opioids are carefully titrated to control pain in terminally ill patients, there is no one maximal dose.

Opioids ≠ Ineffective by Mouth

Oral opioids are very effective analgesics for most patients until swallowing becomes difficult. When prescribing oral morphine, physicians need to remember it is one-third as potent as parenteral morphine. Effective doses must be ordered.

Opioids ≠ Nausea

Nausea is a common physiologic response to opioids and may be experienced by up to 30% of patients when therapy is first begun. When patients have experienced bouts of nausea associated with codeine or morphine, they may believe that they are allergic to opioids, but this is almost never the case. The appropriate action is to prescribe a lower starting dose of the opioid and to order an antiemetic, which can often be withdrawn after several days or weeks with no return of the nausea. Prescribing a different opioid such as oxycodone or hydromorphone is another good alternative. Patients who have been taking regular doses of opioids such as oxycodone or hydrocodone rarely experience nausea when they are switched to morphine. See "Anticipate Problems with Opioid Treatment" on page 35.

Opioids ≠ Euphoria

Opioids do not cause euphoria in terminally ill patients; however, a patient's mood may improve if relief from pain results in a good night's sleep. In hospice/palliative care settings, boosts in mood are more likely to be caused by steroids, dronabinol (Marinol), and methylphenidate (Ritalin).

Use Effective Opioid Dosing

When nonopioid analgesics such as acetaminophen or NSAIDs no longer control pain, the appropriate action usually is to prescribe opioids. Opioids are the safest and most effective agents for most types of cancer-related pain; however, they are effective only when prescribed in effective doses.

Follow WHO Analgesia Ladder

The World Health Organization (WHO) recommends a simple and effective three-step approach for treating pain based on its severity, i.e., mild, mild to moderate, or moderate to severe. The three-step ladder (see Figure 1 on page 28) provides effective pain relief for more than 90% of patients with cancer.[14]

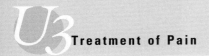

Figure 1: World Health Organization's Analgesic Ladder

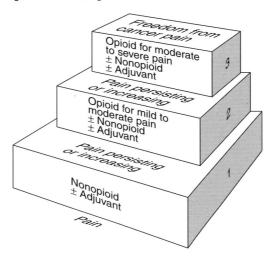

Reproduced by permission of WHO, from *Cancer Pain Relief,* 2nd ed. Geneva, World Health Organization, 1996.

Climbing each step of the ladder sequentially is not necessary. Severe pain mandates the immediate use of opioids for moderate-to-severe pain without progressing sequentially from Step 1 to Step 3. NSAIDs or acetaminophen are recommended for all steps of the ladder. Adjuvant medications can be used at any step to enhance pain relief or to counteract the adverse effects of medications.

- **Step 1:** Step 1 recommends the use of acetaminophen, aspirin, or other nonsteroidal antiinflammatory agents (NSAIDs) to control mild pain.

- **Step 2:** When pain persists, increases, or is mild to moderate, Step 2 is to *add* an opioid such as codeine, hydrocodone, or morphine to the NSAID. At Step 2, fixed-dose combinations of an opioid with acetaminophen or aspirin often are used because combining the drugs provides additive analgesia. When higher doses of an opioid are needed, separate-dosage forms of the opioid and nonopioid are used to avoid the adverse side effects of high-dose acetaminophen and other NSAIDs. When Step 2 is initiated, medications for persistent pain are administered on an around-the-clock basis, with additional as-needed booster doses to control breakthrough pain.

■ **Step 3:** When pain persists, increases, or initially presents as moderate to severe, opioids such as morphine, hydromorphone (Dilaudid), or fentanyl are needed. Patients presenting with moderate to severe pain when first seen by the clinician usually are started at Step 2 or 3 of the ladder.[1]

NOTE: Adjuvant drugs may be used at any step to (1) enhance analgesia, (2) treat concurrent symptoms that exacerbate pain, and (3) provide independent analgesia for specific types of pain. Adjuvant drugs are medications that have analgesic properties for specific types of pain even though they are not usually thought of as pain relievers. Examples of adjuvant drugs include antidepressants used to alleviate neuropathic pain and anticholinergics used to help to control visceral pain. See "Use Adjuvant Drugs when Necessary" on page 40.

The five basic concepts of the WHO ladder for controlling pain are:

1. By the mouth
2. By the clock
3. By the ladder
4. For the individual
5. With attention to detail

Calculate Oral Morphine Equivalents

When pain persists or a different opioid formulation is needed, the easiest way to calculate the required potency is to first convert the opioid to its oral morphine equivalent. Using this method, a physician can compare potencies and order effective doses of medication. Table 2 illustrates oral morphine equivalents.

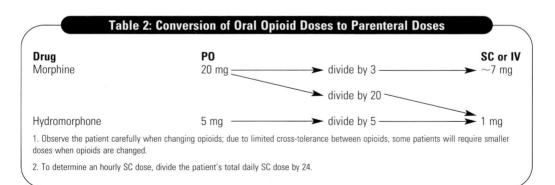

Table 2: Conversion of Oral Opioid Doses to Parenteral Doses

Drug	PO		SC or IV
Morphine	20 mg	divide by 3	~7 mg
		divide by 20	
Hydromorphone	5 mg	divide by 5	1 mg

1. Observe the patient carefully when changing opioids; due to limited cross-tolerance between opioids, some patients will require smaller doses when opioids are changed.

2. To determine an hourly SC dose, divide the patient's total daily SC dose by 24.

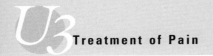

Examples

- A patient who is taking 2 oxycodone 5 mg plus acetaminophen (Percocet) tablets obtains good pain relief, but begins to have difficulty swallowing. As shown in Table 2, 10 mg of oxycodone has the same potency as 15 mg of oral morphine. Because the patient's pain is relieved for 4 hours with 10 mg of oxycodone, an order for an equivalent amount of oral morphine, 15 mg of oral morphine every 4 hours, should continue to provide effective pain relief.

- When difficulty with swallowing occurs, soluble tablets may be an alternative. They dissolve in water (or in the mouth) in about 30 seconds and are inexpensive, are easy to count, and can be taken orally or sublingually. An example is Solutab, a very small soluble tablet made by Eli Lilly. For more information on the use of soluble tablets, concentrated solutions, and rectal preparations, see "Reassess Need for Alternative Routes of Drug Administration" on page 59.

- If 2 tablets of codeine 30 mg or 2 hydrocodone 5-mg tablets are not providing good pain relief for 4 hours, prescribe 1 oxycodone 5-mg tablet every 4 hours. When 2 oxycodone 5-mg tablets no longer provide 4 hours of pain relief, prescribe 15 to 20 mg of oral morphine every 4 hours.

Calculate Injectable Morphine Equivalents

When patients can no longer swallow oral medications, continuous subcutaneous infusion (SC) or intravenous (IV) delivery are effective alternative routes of medication administration and may be required. Intramuscular injections are painful and usually unnecessary. To calculate effective parenteral doses, begin with oral morphine equivalents.

The following method is recommended for converting oral morphine to an equivalent IV or SC dose of morphine:

1. Calculate the patient's total daily requirement of oral morphine.
2. Divide that dose by 3 to determine the patient's total daily requirement of subcutaneous morphine.

The following method is recommended for converting oral morphine to an equivalent dose of IV or SC hydromorphone (Dilaudid):

1. Calculate the patient's total daily requirement of oral morphine.
2. Divide that dose by 20 to determine the patient's total daily dose of SC hydromorphone (Dilaudid).

NOTE: When converting oral hydromorphone to SC hydromorphone, divide the oral dose by 5. For more information about subcutaneous delivery, see "Reassess Need for Alternative Routes of Drug Administration" on page 59.

Use Limited Cross-tolerance Effectively

Over time, a patient receiving treatment with an opioid may experience more effective analgesia from a lower-than-equivalent dose of another opioid. This phenomenon, referred to as *limited cross-tolerance*, also can be utilized when patients experience unacceptable side effects associated with opioid treatment. Often, the side effects can be reduced by *rotating* from one opioid to a less-than-equivalent dose of another.

Use Effective Starting Doses of Opioids

The appropriate starting dose of morphine depends on the following:

- Patient's age, body weight, and degree of cachexia
- Total daily dose of previous analgesics
- Frequency and severity of pain

When initiating opioid therapy, the best policy is to begin with a low dose of an immediate-release product (see Table 3) and then rapidly titrate upward until relief is achieved. (See "Titrate Opioids" on page 33). Slow-release tablets or patches should not be used for rapid dose titration.

Morphine doses can be increased by 30% to 100% or more each day as needed until pain is relieved. Except for slow-release tablets or patches, the opioid should be prescribed every 4 hours on a regular schedule; however, a double dose at bedtime may last 8 hours and allows uninterrupted sleep. Instruct the patient to take an additional dose when breakthrough pain occurs. See "Titrate Opioids" on page 33.

Table 3: Starting Doses for Opioid-Naive Patients		
Infant or child (with mild pain and great concern about side effects)	Child with moderate to severe pain, or adult <60 kg, or elderly patient, or adult with mild pain	Adult>60 kg (with moderate to severe pain and fear that pain will never be relieved)
Start with: <2 mg oral morphine equivalent every 4 hours	**Start with:** 2 to 5 mg oral morphine equivalent every 4 h, e.g., 1/2 to 1 oxycodone and acetaminophen (Percocet) q 4 h	**Start with:** 5 to 10 mg oral morphine equivalent every 4 h, e.g., 1/2 to 1 morphine 10-mg soluble tablet q 4 h

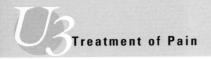

Table 4: Initial Oral Opioid Doses for Children

<50 kilograms and >6 months
0.5 to 1 mg/kg every 3 to 4 hours of codeine
0.2 mg/kg every 3 to 4 hours of oxycodone
0.3 mg/kg every 3 to 4 hours of morphine
0.06 mg/kg every 3 to 4 hours of hydromorphone

<6 Months
Begin with one-quarter to one-third of the above doses and rapidly titrate to effect.

Special Populations

Children, the frail elderly, and patients with HIV disease present special pain-management challenges that often result in gross undertreatment of their pain. Careful assessments and effective doses of medication are particularly important with these populations.

Infants and Children

The high-dose chemotherapy agents used to treat cancer in infants and children often result in treatment-related conditions such as neuropathies, mouth ulcers, and joint pain that may cause more pain than the disease itself, particularly in the case of leukemia. When caring for children, adequately assessing and treating treatment-related sources of pain often is as important as adequately controlling cancer-related pain.

When treating opioid-responsive pain in children, see Table 4. Start with the recommended doses (usually of codeine or hydrocodone) and rapidly titrate to effect, which often results in doses several times larger than the starting dose. See UNIPAC 8.

Frail Elderly

When treating frail elderly patients, begin with half of the usual adult opioid dose and rapidly titrate the dose to effect.

Patients with HIV Disease

Some HIV patients have a history of recreational drug use, which can complicate pain management, but this does not obviate the need to prescribe adequate dosages of opioids and other analgesics.

Because patients with HIV disease may have contracted their disease from drug abuse-related behavior, physicians frequently are reticent to prescribe opioids because of concerns about drug misuse. Such concerns can result in gross undertreatment of HIV patients who are experiencing very high levels of pain. It is easy to confuse a patient's drug-seeking request for stronger doses of medication with a request for relief from uncontrolled pain, careful assessment can help establish reliable reports of pain and provide physician reassurance that appropriate opioid doses are being prescribed. See "Assess for Multiple Causes of Pain" on page 17 and UNIPAC Seven.

When treating pain in this patient population, remember:

- It is easy to confuse requests for drugs that result from undertreatment of pain with requests related to the drug-seeking behavior of addiction.

- Careful assessments can help provide reliable reports of pain.

- Treating pain in the drug-abusing population presents special challenges, but it can be done.[15]

- Pain frequently is undertreated in the HIV population.

- Physicians can set medication limits while making sure that adequate doses are prescribed.

- Information is available on controlling pain in the drug-abusing patient.[16]

- Patients with histories of drug abuse also experience high levels of disease-related pain and should be treated.

Titrate Opioids

Because cancer pain usually increases over time, titrating opioids to provide effective individualized doses is an important pain management technique that is used daily in hospice/palliative care settings. There is no ceiling or maximal recommended opioid dose; large doses of morphine, e.g., several hundred milligrams every 4 hours, may be needed to relieve severe pain.

During the titration process, the physician must remember that immediate-release morphine is a 4-hour drug that reaches its peak effect in approximately 45 to 60 minutes when delivered orally and in about 10 to 20 minutes when delivered subcutaneously. When pain is not relieved within peak times of a higher dose, an additional dose should be given. During the titration process, no ceiling exists on the number of times that a dose may be titrated. Over a 24-hour period, some patients may require more than a 100% increase over their initial daily baseline dose. See Table 5 and "Breakthrough Pain" on page 34.

CAAHPM

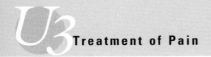

Table 5: Titration Increments for Opioid Dosing*	
Baseline 4-Hour Dose	Titration Increment (~1/2 of 4-Hour dose)
1–10 mg	1–5 mg
10–20 mg	5–10 mg
20–30 mg	10–15 mg
40–50 mg	20–25 mg
100 mg	30–50 mg
200 mg	50–100 mg
500 mg	100–250 mg
1,000 mg	250–500 mg

*These increment doses are also appropriate for use as booster doses. See Breakthrough Pain on page 34.

NOTE: During the entire titration process, continuing reassessment is needed to identify the following:

- Pain that does not respond to opioids may need to be treated with adjuvant drugs or other specific remedies. See page 40.

- Nonphysical pain that must be treated with compassionate listening and involvement of other members of the interdisciplinary team. See *UNIPAC Two: Alleviating Psychological and Spiritual Pain in the Terminally Ill.*

Prevent Breakthrough Pain

Because breakthrough pain is a common problem for many patients, additional opioid doses should be prescribed on an as-needed basis. These additional opioid doses (referred to as *booster* doses because they boost the analgesic level) should be approximately one-half the regular 4-hour opioid dose, or about 10% of the 24-hour dose. Regular use of additional doses (more than 3 to 4 times daily) may signal the need to increase the baseline dose and/or the need for a co-analgesic. See Table 5 for examples of appropriate booster doses.

Avoid Certain Drugs and Routes

Although there are many exceptions, Table 6 describes drugs and medication delivery routes that should be avoided in hospice/palliative care settings.

Table 6: Drugs and Routes to Avoid in Hospice/Palliative Care Settings

Drugs

Meperidine (Demerol)	Very low potency. Toxic metabolite accumulation.
Pentazocine (Talwin)	No more potent than codeine. High incidence of hallucinations and agitation (30% in cancer patients). Inhibits analgesia of morphine.

Routes

IM injections	Morphine 30 mg PO is as potent as 10 mg IM/SC. Avoid the pain and expense of IM injections with PO or SL morphine. If patient cannot tolerate anything PO, start a SC infusion or give slow-release morphine tablets rectally.

Anticipate Problems with Opioid Treatment

Patient Compliance

In most cases, patient compliance improves when physicians take time to listen carefully to the patient's and family's concerns and provide further education about opioid use and treatable side effects. Patient and family concerns about opioid use are often based on misconceptions. Compliance problems also arise from conditions such as swallowing difficulties, concerns about opioid-related constipation, and lack of patient access to expensive medications.

Adverse Side Effects

Common adverse side effects include constipation, nausea, sedation/drowsiness, confusion, and hallucinations. Less common side effects include urinary retention (which can result from constipation-related impactions) and myoclonic jerks. Side effects are dose related and may be specific to a particular drug. With the exception of constipation, most side effects can be managed by rotating to another opioid or by adding an adjuvant analgesic, which allows for a reduction in the opioid dose.

Constipation. Most patients in hospice/palliative care settings require a maintenance laxative regimen to prevent and/or relieve constipation, a symptom commonly experienced by terminally ill patients due to the following:

- Low fluid intake

- Impaired mobility

- Complicating medical conditions, such as bowel obstructions and hemorrhoids

- Drug therapies that impair gut motility

Constipation is such a common side effect of opioid use that nearly all patients receiving opioid therapy should be placed on regular doses of laxatives to prevent its distressing symptoms. A combination of a softening agent and a stimulant laxative should be used, and dosages should be increased as opioid doses increase. Effective prevention requires constant vigilance and awareness of the physiological and social components of constipation.

Assessment of Constipation

On admission, each patient should be carefully assessed for constipation. The assessment should include:

- Step 1: A detailed bowel history that includes information on:
    a. Stool frequency and consistency
    b. Previous laxative use and its effectiveness
    c. Associated problems, such as lack of privacy or long distances to the toilet
- Step 2: Abdominal examination
- Step 3: Rectal exam, if indicated

Impaction Removal

- Hard impaction: If a hard fecal impaction is found, digital removal should follow fecal softening with an oil-retention enema and perhaps premedication with diazepam or midazolam.
- Soft impaction: Soft impactions may respond to bisacodyl suppositories or large-volume tap water or phosphate enemas.

To prevent recurrence of constipation, the removal of hard and soft impactions must be followed with a vigorous laxative protocol that includes both stool softeners and stimulant agents such as senna or bisacodyl with docusate.

Suggested Laxative Regimen

Patients with a history of constipation may wish to continue using whichever laxative has produced results in the past. Avoid bulk-forming agents such as psyllium or methylcellulose because they tend to form impactions when patients can no longer take adequate amounts of fluids.

Patients with no previous history of constipation can try the following:

- Docusate (Colace) or
- Docusate with casanthranol or a similar gentle laxative

Table 7: An Effective Stepwise Laxative Regimen		
Step	**Medication**	**Dose**
1	Docusate (100 mg)	1 cap BID
2	Senna (Senokot) or bisacodyl (Dulcolax)	1 tab QD
3	Senna or bisacodyl	1 tab BID
4	Senna or bisacodyl	2 tabs BID
5	Senna or bisacodyl	3 tabs BID
6	Senna	4 tabs BID
	plus sorbitol	15 cc BID
7	Senna	To 4 tabs BID
	plus sorbitol	30 cc BID
8	Senna	4 tabs BID
	plus sorbitol	30 cc TID-QID

Note: One generic senna tablet 187 mg ~ senna extract 5 mg (Senokot).

Most patients require individually titrated doses of potent bowel stimulants, such as the following:

- Senna (Senokot), or

- Bisacodyl (Dulcolax)

As with opioid therapy, the most effective laxative regimen for the control and prevention of constipation is one that follows a stepwise approach and is ongoing, instead of being administered on an as-needed basis. (See Table 7 for an example of an effective, step-wise laxative regimen.)

The physician must specify the initial laxative regimen step on admission orders (e.g., senna 5 mg PO BID) and specify that an ongoing laxative regimen must be instituted. If the patient has not had a bowel movement in 2 days, the laxative dose should be increased to the next level. If the patient has not had a bowel movement in 3 days, one of the following treatments should be given once or twice daily until results are obtained:

- Digital disimpaction followed by 2 bisacodyl suppositories, or

- Sodium phosphate 30 cc PO repeated in 2 hours if needed, or

- Mineral oil or soapsuds enema

After successful treatment, the patient should resume the step-wise regimen at the level at which the above treatment was initiated. If none of the treatments is effective, the physician must reassess the situation and initiate appropriate therapy.

AAHPM

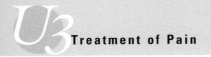

Severe Constipation

Rectal suppositories and enemas rarely are needed when a laxative regimen is conscientiously followed. However, if severe constipation develops, it should be treated vigorously. The following treatments are suggested:

- Sodium phosphate: some patients prefer a purgative dose of a saline laxative, such as sodium phosphate (Fleet Phospho-Soda), but it can cause cramping and bloating. Use 30 mL at a time PO every 2 hours.

- Bisacodyl 10-mg suppositories (1 or 2 PR) often are effective in 15 minutes to an hour.

- Soapsuds or phosphate enemas occasionally may be required.

- Higher-volume enemas can increase efficacy.

- Sometimes, when nothing else works, a milk and molasses enema can be effective. Add 1 cup of powdered milk and 1 cup of molasses or corn syrup to a liter of warm water and administer rectally.

Special Situations

- Bowel obstruction: Patients who continue to pass some stool through their obstruction may benefit from a softening agent, such as higher-dose docusate or low-dose sorbitol. Due to the obstruction, other patients probably will vomit one or two times a day, but they can be kept comfortable on a SC infusion of an opioid and antiemetic. See *UNIPAC Four: Management of Selected Nonpain Symptoms in the Terminally Ill.*

- Colicky abdominal pains: Pain can be minimized with careful dose titration and/or the addition of docusate or sorbitol for stool softening. Doses of up to 300 mg of docusate tid or 30 mL of sorbitol tid are not unusual.

- Stimulation alone is ineffective or poorly tolerated: Osmotic agents, such as sorbitol or lactulose (Chronulac) 10 g/15 mL (15 to 60 mL bid-tid), can be effective. *Note:* Sorbitol is less expensive, equally effective, and less nauseating than lactulose.[17]

- Opioid bowel syndrome: Patients receiving opioid analgesics may develop opioid bowel syndrome, which resembles bowel obstruction. Metoclopramide (either PO or by SC infusion) can provide relief.

Social and Psychological Aspects of Constipation

The social and psychological aspects of constipation can interfere with its treatment and prevention. Attention must be paid to:

- Privacy needs: A private commode with easy access is essential.

- Acceptable caregivers: Patients may not allow opposite-sex relatives or caretakers to give them suppositories or enemas.

- Cost issues: The high cost of some laxatives can interfere with compliance.

Nausea and Vomiting. When opioids are first prescribed, they may induce nausea and vomiting in 10% to 40% of patients. Because patients frequently believe nausea and vomiting indicate an allergic response to an opioid, care should be taken to explain that such symptoms are dose-related, temporary side effects, not allergies.

When morphine is prescribed before another opioid such as oxycodone has been used, order an antiemetic such as prochlorperazine (Compazine) or transdermal scopolamine (Transderm Scop) for a few days to prevent nausea and vomiting. Usually, the antiemetic can be phased out after several days or weeks. Nausea or vomiting is less likely to occur if the patient has been taking regular doses of other opioids before starting morphine, so consider using hydrocodone or oxycodone first, if practical. For other causes and suggested treatments on nausea and vomiting, see *UNIPAC Four: Management of Selected Nonpain Symptoms in the Terminally Ill.*

Sedation, Drowsiness, and Somnolence. When opioid therapy is initiated, temporary sedation frequently occurs, but it usually clears within 2 to 5 days after achieving a steady dose of effective analgesia. Although opioids directly affect the central nervous system, accumulated exhaustion and sleep deprivation caused by uncontrolled pain usually are the major contributing factors to somnolence. When pain relief is achieved, the patient finally may be able to sleep for long periods of time.

Continued drowsiness may indicate a need to decrease the opioid dose or change to a less sedating co-analgesic, but it may also be a sign of disease progression. Such sedation is not an indication for the use of naloxone (Narcan). If drowsiness remains troublesome, try decreasing the opioid dose and adding a nonsedating co-analgesic like a NSAID. Rotation of the opioid (i.e., morphine to hydromorphone or oxycodone) may accomplish pain relief with lower, less sedating doses. A few patients will benefit from the addition of an amphetamine such as methylphenidate (Ritalin) 5 to 15 mg in the early morning and at noon.

Confusion, Hallucinations, and Cognitive Impairment. Opioids may cause or aggravate confusion and hallucinations in a small number of patients, especially the elderly. If this occurs, switch to a different opioid at a lower dose, if possible. Confusion also may result from brain metastases, hepatic, renal or respiratory insufficiency, or other metabolic changes associated with advancing disease. The addition of haloperidol or a phenothiazine such as thioridazine (Mellaril) may be necessary to calm the patient when confusion cannot be reversed. See *UNIPAC Four: The Management of Selected Nonpain Symptoms in the Terminally Ill.*

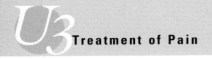

Opioid Overdose

Opioid overdose is rare when titration procedures are followed correctly; however, it can occur and should be suspected when levels of consciousness and respirations decrease concomitantly, particularly when respirations decrease to <6 per minute in the presence of myoclonic twitching, constricted pupils, skeletal muscle flaccidity, and cold or clammy skin.

If the patient is drowsy and breathing slowly, stop administering opioids for a while and simply wait for the drug to wear off. Opioids can usually then be restarted at a lower dose. When administration of naloxone is necessary, do not follow the PDR recommendations, which may cause a traumatic return of agonizing pain. Instead, dilute 1 amp (0.4 mg) of naloxone in 10 mL of saline and give 1 mL of this diluted mixture (0.04 mg) IV every 5 minutes until partial reversal occurs. Repeating the process may be necessary because naloxone has a shorter half-life than most opioids.

Use Adjuvant Drugs When Necessary

Several types of drugs not usually thought of as analgesics are referred to as co-analgesics or adjuvant drugs because they effectively relieve certain types of pain that do not respond fully to opioid therapy. As with opioids, adjuvant drugs often must be titrated to manage pain effectively (e.g., increased doses of antidepressants or anticonvulsants may be needed to manage neuropathic pain effectively, and increased doses of anticholinergics may be needed to manage visceral pain effectively).

Patients with Liver Disease

Changes in drug disposition reflect the liver's degree of impairment (i.e., alcoholic liver disease can range from fatty liver, with little change in the disposition of most drugs, to severe cirrhosis, with major changes in the disposition of certain classes of drugs). Hepatic neoplasms also show variability in the effect of drug disposition, depending on type (primary versus secondary), size, invasiveness, and vascularity of the tumor mass. Dispositional changes associated with liver that require alterations in a normal drug regimen are determined by a drug's dispositional characteristics and the biologic determinants of the system. In patients with liver disease, the degree of hepatic metabolism is not solely responsible for needed dosage adjustments. Lipid-soluble drugs have a large volume of distribution and require metabolism into more water-soluble moieties. In advanced disease, albumin levels decrease with advanced nutritional impairment; therefore, protein-bound drugs increase the drug's apparent volume of distribution. Liver disease has the greatest effect on drugs that undergo extensive oxidative metabolism.

Liver disease should have no effect on the disposition of drugs excreted unchanged by the kidneys. No useful noninvasive test of liver function exists to guide dosage adjustments. Typical liver function tests reflect but do not predict the extent of liver damage.

Table 8: Examples of Dosage Adjustments in Patients with Liver Disease[18,19]

Medication Adjuvants	Hepatic Elimination	Dosage Adjustment
Cabamazepine	>98% hepatic	Decrease dose
Dexamethasone	>97% hepatic	Decrease dose
Phenytoin	>95% hepatic	Decrease dose in severe disease
Mexiletine	90% hepatic	Decrease dose 60–70%
Prednisone	>85% hepatic	None
Analgesics		
Acetaminophen	>95% hepatic	Avoid chronic use*
Fentanyl	92% hepatic	None
Ibuprofen	>99% hepatic	Decrease dose in severe disease*
Methadone	80% hepatic	None or decrease*
Morphine	90% GI and hepatic	Decrease dose or use a different opioid
Naproxyn	>90% hepatic	Decrease dose in severe disease
Propoxyphene	>95% GI and hepatic	Decrease by 50%*
Antidepressants		
Amitriptyline	Primarily hepatic	Decrease by 50%
Fluoxetine	Primarily hepatic	Decrease by 50%
Nefazodone	Primarily hepatic	Decrease dose
Antiemetics		
Metoclopramide	80% hepatic	Decrease by 50%
Ondansetron	>95% hepatic	Decrease frequency in severe disease
Antihistamine		
Diphenhydramine	>98% hepatic	Decrease dose
Anxiolytics		
Alprazolam	>90% hepatic	Decrease by 50%
Chlordiazepoxide	>99% hepatic	Decrease*
Diazepam	>97% hepatic	Chronic, decrease dose
Lorazepam	>98% hepatic	None
Midazolam	>95% hepatic	Decrease dose by 50%
Diuretics		
Bumetanide	36% hepatic	None
Furosemide	35% hepatic	None
Hydrochlorothiazide	<10% hepatic	None
Spironolactone	>85% hepatic	None
Triamterene	>95% hepatic	Decrease dose

(*Continued*)

Gastrointestinal		
Cimetidine	40% hepatic	Decrease dose in severe disease
Famotidine	30% hepatic	None
Omeprazole	>90% hepatic	Decrease dose by 50%
Ranitidine	30% hepatic	None
Sedative/Hypnotics		
Temazepam	>98% hepatic	None
Other		
Pamidronate	30% hepatic	None

*In hepatic failure, choose an alternative agent.

Patients with Renal Failure

In patients with advanced disease, renal problems can result from a variety of conditions, including hypovolemia, diminished cardiac function, primary renal diseases, vasculitis, hypotension, allergic reactions, intratubular deposition or post-renal obstructive problems. Because many medications and their metabolites are metabolized and/or excreted by the kidneys, individualized pharmacologic dosing is important in patients with renal impairment. Renal failure can also contribute to the development of electrolyte, acid–base, vascular volume, nutritional and hematologic problems. Renal failure can either increase or decrease the volume of distribution of certain drugs, thus effecting their metabolism. Acid-base changes occurring with renal failure can effect protein binding; thus altering bound and unbound levels of medications and their metabolites. Be aware of age-related declines in renal function in the elderly (see Table 9).

Measurements of creatinine clearance (CL_{CR}) are helpful when determining appropriate medication dosing in patients with renal disease. The following are easy methods for estimating creatinine clearance:

- For males: $CL_{CR} = (140 - age) \times$ weight (in kilograms) divided by $72 \times$ serum creatinine
- For females: $CL_{CR} = CL_{CR}$ male $\times 0.85$

Bone or Soft Tissue Pain: Corticosteroids/NSAIDs

Bone pain requires a particularly careful assessment.[23] If there is severe pain on weight bearing, a radiograph may reveal a potential for pathologic fracture for which orthopedic stabilization or radiation therapy may be needed. Spinal cord compression occurs in about 5% of cancer patients, and local or radicular (neuropathic) pain may be the only sign before the development of paralysis.[24] Back pain associated with paresthesia, sen-

Table 9: Examples of Dosage Adjustments for Patients with Renal Failure[20,21,22]

Medication	Adjustment for Renal Failure (CLCR)	
	10–50 mL/min	<10 mL/min
Adjuvants		
Amitriptyline	100%	100%
Carbamazepine	100%	100%
Desipramine	100%	100%
Dexamethasone	100%	100%
Mexiletine	100%	50%–75%
Nortriptyline	100%	100%
Phenytoin	100%	100%
Prednisone	100%	100%
Gabapentin	q 12–24 h	qod
Analgesics		
Acetaminophen	q 6 h dosing	q 8 h dosing
Acetylsalicylate*	q 4-6 h dosing	Avoid
Codeine	75%	50%
Diclofenac*	25%–50%	25%
Fentanyl	100%	100%
Ibuprofen*	100%	100%
Ketorolac*	50%	25%–50%
Methadone	100%	50%–75%
Morphine	75%	50%
Naproxen*	100%	100%
Propoxyphene	100%	Avoid
Sulindac*	100%	100%
Antidepressants		
Amoxapine	100%	100%
Bupropion	100%	100%
Fluoxetine	100%	100%
Sertraline	100%	100%
Antiemetics		
Cisapride	100%	50%
Haloperidol	100%	100%
Granisetron	100%	100%
Metoclopramide	75%	50%
Ondansetron	100%	100%
Prochlorperazine	100%	100%

(*Continued*)

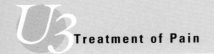

Medication	Adjustment for Renal Failure (CLCR)	
	10–50 mL/min	<10 mL/min
Antihistamines		
Diphenhydramine	100%	100%
Hydroxyzine	50%	50%
Anxiolytics		
Alprazolam	100%	100%
Chlordiazepoxide	100%	50%
Clonazepam	100%	100%
Diazepam	100%	100%
Midazolam	100%	50%
Oxazepam	100%	100%
Bronchodilators (oral)		
Albuterol	75%	50%
Terbutaline	50%	Avoid
Theophylline	100%	100%
Diuretics		
Bumetadine	100%	100%
Furosemide	100%	100%
Spironolactone	q 12–24 h dosing	Avoid
Thiazides	100%	Avoid
Triamterene	q 12 h dosing	Avoid
Gastrointestinal		
Cimetidine	50%–75%	25%–50%
Famotidine	25%–50%	10%
Misoprostol	100%	100%
Omeprazole	100%	100%
Ranitidine	50%	25%
Sucralfate	Avoid	Avoid
Hypoglycemic Agents		
Acarbose	Avoid	Avoid
Glipizide	50%	50%
Glyburide	100%	100%
Insulin	75%	50%
Inotropic Agents		
Dobutamine	100%	100%
Milrinone	100%	50%–75%

Sedative/Hypnotics

Flurazepam	100%	100%
Phenobarbitol	100%	100%
Temazepam	100%	100%
Triazolam	100%	100%

Other

Chlorpromazine	100%	100%
Warfarin	100%	100%

100% means no dosage adjustment required.

*NSAIDs can decrease glomerular filtration and precipitate renal failure in a patient with renal insufficiency.

sory deficit, or bowel or bladder incontinence in an ambulatory patient who is a candidate for surgery or radiotherapy should signal an evaluation for spinal cord compression by spinal imaging.

Continuous bone pain may respond well to opioids alone, but if side effects are dose limiting, the addition of a NSAID (in full antiarthritic doses) or a steroid can be effective. See Table 10. If one NSAID is not effective, switching to a different NSAID may be. The analgesia and toxicity of NSAID are dose related. Dyspepsia is not a reliable

Table 10: NSAIDs and Other Analgesics

Generic Name	Approx. half-life (h)	Dosing Schedule (h)	Starting Dose (mg/day)[1,2] Adults >50 kg	Maximum Dose (mg/day)[1]	Excretion	Comments
Para-aminophenol Derivatives						
Acetaminophen (Tylenol)[2]	2–4	q 4–6	2,600	4,000	85% renal	Lacks peripheral anti-inflammatory and anti-platelet effect. Excessive dosing → liver toxicity. Monitor platelet and liver function with chronic disease. Adults and children >50 kg: 10–15 mg/kg q 4 h.

(*Continued*)

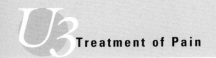

Nonsteroidal Antiinflammatory Analgesics

Generic Name	Approx. half-life (h)	Dosing Schedule (h)	Starting Dose (mg/day)[1] Adults >50 kg	Maximum Dose (mg/day)[1]	Excretion	Comments
Salicylates						
Acetylsalicylic acid (aspirin)[3]	3–12	q 4–6	3,750	6,000	100% renal	May inhibit platelet aggregation for >1 week. Contraindicated in children with fever or other viral syndromes.
Choline magnesium trisalicylate (Trilisate)[2,3]	8–12	8–12	Initial dose: 1,500 mg; then 1,500 mg q 8–12 h	4,500	100% renal	Approved for children. Minimal GI toxicity. Suspension available.
Diflunisal (Dolobid)[3]	8–12	12	Initial dose: 1,000 mg; then 500 mg q 12 h	1,000	90% renal, <5% fecal	—
Salsalate (Disalcid)[2,3]	8–12	12	Initial dose: 1,500 mg; then 1,500 mg q 12 h	3,000	100% renal	—
Propionic Acids						
Flurbiprofen (Ansaid)[3]	5–6	8–12	100	300	65–85% renal	—
Ibuprofen (Motrin), Advil (Nuprin)[3]	2–4	4–8	400–600 mg q 6–8 h	3,200	50–75% renal	Suspension formulation available.
Ketoprofen (Orudis)[3]	2–4	6–8	25–50 mg q 8 h in mild renal impairment and elderly. 75 mg q 8 h or 50 mg q 6 h	300	50–90% renal, 1–8% fecal	—
Naproxen (Naprosyn)[3]	13	12	500	1,500	95% renal	Cautious use of >1,500 mg/day may be more efficacious. Suspension available.

Naproxen sodium (Anaprox, Alleve)[3]	13	12	550	1,100	95% renal	—
Oxaprozin (Daypro)[3]	50–60; 40 with repeated dosing	24	1,200	1,800	60% renal, 30–35% fecal	—
Acetic Acids						
Diclofenac (Voltaren)[3]	2	6	100	200	50–70% renal, 30–35% fecal	—
Indomethacin (Indocin, Indocide, Indomethine)[3]	4–5	8–24	75	200	60% renal, 30% fecal	Available in sustained release and rectal formulations. Greater GI and CNS toxicity.
Sulindac (Clinoril)[3]	8–16	12	300	400	50% renal, 25% fecal	—
Tolmetin (Tolectin)[3]	1	8	1,200	1,800	100% renal	—
Oxicam						
Piroxicam (Feldene)[3]	50	25	20	40	67% renal, 33% fecal	Progressive increase in response may occur because of long half-life. Steady state 7–12 days after initiation of therapy.
Fenamates						
Meclofenamic acid (Meclomen)[3]	50 mins–3.3 h	4–6	50–100	400	67% renal, 20–25% fecal	Dose-related diarrhea.
Mefenamic acid (Ponstel)[3]	2	6	Loading dose: 500 mg; then 250 mg	1,000	67% renal, 33% fecal	Intended for short-term use. Dose-related diarrhea.
COX-2 Inhibitors						
Celecoxib (Celebrex)[2,3]	11	12	100 mg bid	400	97% hepatic metabolism 3% renal	Less GI toxicity. Higher cost.
Rofecoxib (Vioxx)[2,3]	17	24	12.5	50	99% hepatic metabolism 1% renal	Less GI toxicity. Higher cost.

(*Continued*)

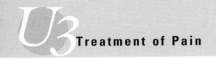

Generic Name	Approx. half-life (h)	Dosing Schedule (h)	Starting Dose (mg/day)[1] Adults >50 kg	Maximum Dose (mg/day)[1]	Excretion	Comments
Pyrrolopyrrole						
Ketorolac (Toradol)[3]	4–6	4–6	IV/IM 30–60 mg loading dose; then 1/2 loading dose q 6 h; PO 10 mg q 6 h	120 mg IV/IM; 40 mg PO	91% renal, 6% fecal	Short-term use only (5 days).
Pyranocarboxylic Acids						
Etodolac (Lodine)[3]	6–7	6–8	200–400	1,200	60% renal, 27% fecal	
Naphthlalkanones						
Nabumetone (Relafen)[3]	23–30	q 12–24 h	1,000	2,000	renal	A pro-drug. GI and kidney toxicity may be less common.

1. Starting and maximal dosing are not intended to preclude clinical judgment of prescriber. Dosage reduction recommended for elderly, renal insufficiency, multiple medications. Initial doses usually may be titrated upward. Doses can be incremented weekly. Studies of NSAIDs in the cancer population are limited. Dosing guidelines are based on studies in inflammatory diseases, thus doses in cancer patients are empiric.

2. Minimal platelet effects.

3. NSAIDs can cause severe GI and renal toxicities, especially in elderly and chronically ill patients or if prescribed at high dosages over long periods. If they must be used in high risk circumstances, consider regular monitoring of stools for occult blood, BUN, creatinine, and liver function.

predictor of gastric ulceration. Elderly patients, patients requiring steroids, or those with histories of ulcers are at higher risk. Such patients may benefit from a COX-2 inhibitor or addition of misoprostol (Cytotec) 100 to 200 μg to tid-qid.

Bone metastases can cause severe neuropathic pain (see next section) or incident pain. This type of pain is usually much more severe on movement or weight bearing. If radiation or bracing are not desirable or effective, a short-acting opioid such as fentanyl can be given in bolus form by SC injection, oral-transmucosal lozenge, nebulizer, or nasal spray for effective relief.[25]

Other potentially effective adjuvant analgesics for bone pain include calcitonin, radioisotopes, or biphosphonates. (See Table 11.) None of these adjuvants has proved to be

Table 11: Selected Adjuvant Analgesics for Bone Pain

First Line	Examples
■ NSAID with/without misoprostol	■ Naproxen, sulindac
■ Corticosterioid	■ Dexamethasone, prednisone
Second Line	**Examples**
■ Radioisotope	■ Strontium-89, sumarium 153
■ Bisphosphonate	■ Pamidronate, clodronate
■ Calcitonin	■ Nasal or SC salmon calcitonin

more effective than opioids combined with NSAIDS, but they can be useful in some difficult situations.

When NSAIDs are contraindicated because the patient has few platelets (e.g., after chemotherapy or with extensive marrow displacement), a COX-2 inhibitor or a nonacetylated salicylate such as choline magnesium trisalicylate (Trilisate) or salsalate (Disalcid) may provide some analgesia without compromising the functioning of the remaining platelets. Another option is a corticosteroid, such as dexamethasone 4 mg bid PO or SC. As with other NSAIDs, both of these alternatives may cause gastritis or peptic ulcer disease, so consider protecting the stomach with misoprostol or an H2 blocker.

Neuropathic or Nerve Pain: Antidepressants and Anticonvulsants

A thorough neurologic evaluation often can identify specific neurologic pain syndromes.[26] See Table 12. Neurologic pain syndromes usually can also be identified by

Table 12: Neuropathic Cancer Pain Syndromes[26]

■ Cranial neuralgic	■ Peripheral nerve syndromes
■ Leptomeningeal metastases	■ Postsurgical pain syndromes
■ Epidural spinal cord compression	■ Postradiation pain syndromes
■ Lumbosacral or brachial plexopathies	■ Postchemotherapy peripheral neuropathy
■ Polyneuropathies	■ Acute herpetic and postherpetic neuralgias

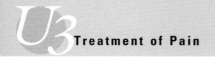

the patient's description of types of pain associated with each syndrome. Pain character-ized as burning, scalding or tingling is associated with continuous dysesthesia. Pain characterized as shooting, grabbing, or stabbing is associated with a lancinating or paroxysmal dysesthesia. If a specific therapy is not available, selection of the most useful adjuvant is based on each drug's indications, likely side effects, potential adverse effects, drug interactions, and dosing guidelines.[27] See Table 13.

Table 13: Selected Adjuvant Analgesics for Neuropathic Pain

Pain Character	Drug Class	Examples	Notes
Continuous burning or tingling, pain on light touch	Tricyclic antidepressants	Amitriptyline (Elavil) 10–50 PO mg qhs	Best studied, sedating, start with low dose, anticholinergic effects.
		Doxepin (Sinequan) 10–50 mg PO qhs	10 mg/cc suspension available. If patient unable to swallow, insert capsules rectally (50 mg q 12 h).
		Trazodone (Desyrel) 25–150 mg PO qhs	Less anticholinergic effect, one-third as potent as amitriptyline, sedating.
		Nortriptyline (Pamelor) 10–50 mg PO qhs	Less anticholinergic effect. Suspension available.
Shooting, stabbing pain	Anticonvulsants	Gabapentin (Neurontin) 100–300 mg PO qhs and increase rapidly as tolerated	Effective but costly.
		Valproic acid (Depakote) 250 mg PO tid-qid	Both carbamazepine and valproic acid are absorbed from the rectum.
		Carbamazepine (Tegretol) 200 mg PO q 6–12 h	Start at lower dose if pain is not severe Liquid form available. If patient unable to swallow, crush tablets, put in gelatin capsules, and give rectally (600 mg q 6–8 h)
		Clonazepam (Klonopin) 0.5 mg PO bid-qid or 0.01 mg/kg initially	Sedating.

	Phenytoin (Dilantin) 300–400 mg PO qd or load with 15–20 mg/kg IV (in a crisis)	Rarely first line.
Local anesthetics	Mexiletine (Mexitil) 150 mg bid-qid or 1 mg/kg in bid-tid doses; may require up to 900 mg/d	GI side effects. Monitor EKG &/or blood levels as appropriate.
	Lidocaine SC or IV infusion	Monitor EKG.
	Lidocaine transdermal 5% (Lidoderm)	Apply to painful areas.
	Lidocaine/prilocaine topical (Emla)	Apply to painful areas.
Other agents	Clonidine 0.1– 0.3 mg PO bid or clonidine transdermal (Catapres–TTS) 0.1–0.3 mg/24 h	Monitor blood pressure, watch for rebound hypertension, depression, bradycardia.
	Baclofen 5–20 mg PO tid	Watch for drowsiness, dizziness.
	Calcitonin nasal spray (Miacalcin)	Delayed onset of analgesia, few side effects.
	Capsaicin topical (Zostrix) 0.025 or 0.075% cream apply tid-qid	Commonly causes burning sensation and thermal hyperalgesia.

An antidepressant and an anticonvulsant may be needed. In difficult cases, check for therapeutic serum levels of both the antidepressant and the anticonvulsant.

The burning, tingling pain of neuropathic pain can be relieved with low to full doses (10 to 100 mg) of a tricyclic antidepressant such as amitriptyline (Elavil), nortriptyline (Pamelor), doxepin (Sinequan), or desipramine (Norpramin). These drugs can also help with insomnia and depression.

When neuropathic pain is characterized by shooting or stabbing pain, consider using anticonvulsants such as gabapentin (Neurontin), carbamazepine (Tegretol), or valproic acid (Depakene). Full anticonvulsant dosages may be required. In difficult cases, check

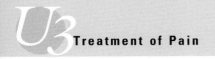

for therapeutic serum levels of both the antidepressant and the anticonvulsant; however, there is no need to check blood levels of gabapentin.

Both an antidepressant and an anticonvulsant are often required.[28] When patients cannot swallow even the liquid forms of doxepin or carbamazepine, insert doxepin capsules rectally (50 mg every 12 hours) and/or crush carbamazepine tablets, put them in gelatin capsules, and give 600 mg rectally every 8 to 12 hours.[29] In addition to antidepressants and anticonvulsants, antiarrhythmics such as lidocaine or mexiletine (Mexitil) and other agents (see Table 13) have alleviated neuropathic pain in some patients.

Raised Intracranial Pressure: Corticosteroids

Dexamethasone 4 mg (or more) PO bid to qid (with an opioid) is the drug of choice to relieve pain caused by raised intracranial pressure in patients whose expected length and quality of life warrant the initiation of corticosteroid therapy. When patients cannot swallow, insert a 25-gauge butterfly needle capped with an injection site into the subcutaneous tissue, secure it, and teach family members to inject the 4 mg per mL dexamethasone into the injection site 2 to 4 times per day. When raised intracranial pressure is associated with a rapid deterioration in the patient's mental status, a large increase in the opioid dose to control headache may be more appropriate than initiating corticosteroid therapy or giving it by injection.

Visceral Pain: Anticholinergics

When cramping, colic-like abdominal pains are not due to urinary retention or fecal impaction, consider using an anticholinergic drug such as oxybutynin (Ditropan) 5 to 10 mg three times a day or hyoscyamine (Levsin) 0.125 mg 1 to 2 PO or SL every 4 hours as needed. Alert the patient to the possibility of increased constipation, dry mouth, or blurred vision. The laxative regimen may need to be increased due to worsened constipation.

If the patient cannot swallow tablets, consider sublingual hyoscyamine (Levsin SL) or transdermal scopolamine (Transderm Scop) and Glycopyrrolate (Robinul) can also be combined with an opioid and given by SC infusion.

Use Nonpharmacological Methods When Appropriate

In hospice/palliative care settings, nonpharmacologic methods of pain control are generally appropriate for use as adjunct therapies to pharmacologic treatment, rather than as stand-alone treatments. The following methods can be invaluable for improving quality of life and enhancing the efficacy of drug therapy:

- Distraction: music, art, movies, reading, books on tape
- Guided imagery or hypnosis
- Progressive relaxation
- Meditation
- Massage therapy
- Transepidural nerve stimulator (TENS)
- Acupuncture

Avoid Placebos

When pain continues to occur in the absence of clinical findings, adequate treatment requires dedication, persistence, and a willingness to consider many treatment modalities. Except in controlled trials with patient consent, the use of placebos to control pain is prohibited by the principles of patient autonomy and informed consent, as well as by the hospice/palliative care commitment to a patient's inclusion as a member of the healthcare team.

Treat Nonphysical Causes of Pain

Emotional, spiritual, and social pain may be caused by conditions such as the following:

- Anxiety
- Depression
- Isolation and loneliness
- Fear
- Financial concerns
- Loss of faith
- Loss of meaning

In hospice/palliative care settings and in this UNIPAC, total pain is described as a combination of the patient's physical, social, emotional, and spiritual pain. Although this model of total pain is helpful for the purposes of emphasizing the multifaceted nature of pain, it has the unfortunate effect of reinforcing the dichotomous view of pain as be-

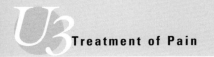

ing either physical or nonphysical. This view tends to diminish the patient's suffering and relegate physicians to the role of mechanical technicians whose only purpose is the manipulation of dosages and dials.

Instead, the concept of pain must be enlarged to include physical distress and suffering, which are phenomenologically distinct. A person may be in severe physical pain but not be suffering because the pain is explainable and has meaning, for instance, the pain of childbirth or kidney stones. However, when the source of pain is unknown and when it is chronic, overwhelming, and without meaning, it generally results in suffering.[30] For more information, see *UNIPAC 2: Alleviating Psychological and Spiritual Pain in the Terminally Ill*.

Suffering: A Definition

Suffering can be defined as "the state of severe distress associated with events that threaten the intactness of the person."[31] Suffering may occur as a result of symptoms such as acute pain or shortness of breath, but it extends beyond the physical. It occurs when patients perceive the impending destruction of their personhood, and it continues until the threat of disintegration has passed or until the patient's integrity can be restored in some way.[32] Patients may experience extreme suffering in the absence of physical pain.

Physician As Healer

In the process of providing relief from suffering, physicians can assume an important and enlarged role, that of healer. When cure is no longer possible, a healing physician assists with the following:

- Lending strength to patients who are suffering not only from the impending loss of all the relationships that they have ever known, but also from the impending loss of all their unrealized hopes and dreams

- Reinforcing new definitions of hope as patients try to come to terms with the regrets of a lifetime

- Helping patients transcend their current physical state by assisting with the search for a broader context of meaning that includes family and community[32]

For patients and other laypersons, the relief of suffering (regardless of its source) is one of the primary goals of medicine. When, during the last days and months of life, the patient's need for healing seems to conflict with the physician's ongoing need to cure, poor communication may be the result. To assume the strength-lending role of healer, physicians must relieve the pain caused by noncancer and cancer-related medical conditions, work closely with the interdisciplinary team, and then remain fully attentive as patients find meaning in their lives.

Alleviating Mild Nonphysical Pain: Social, Emotional, and Spiritual Pain

When assessment indicates the presence of mild nonphysical pain, supportive counseling, nonjudgmental listening, and education often can provide relief. However, to be effective, physicians must be able to discuss these real sources of pain with empathy and compassion.

Alleviating Moderate to Severe Nonphysical Suffering

When more complicated social, emotional, and spiritual issues result in suffering, the physician should consider making referrals to other professionals, such as the patient's religious or spiritual adviser and/or a counselor or social worker with special training in issues related to terminal care. The inclusion of pharmacologic treatment also must be considered when nonphysical pain and suffering result from depression and/or anxiety that:

- Is severe enough to interfere with the patient's ability to function

- Worsens rather than resolves with time

- Persists more than 7 days[33]

Disabling anxiety and depression are not necessary parts of the dying process; any hesitancy to treat them pharmacologically is as misguided as hesitancy to adequately treat cancer-related physical pain. There is accumulating evidence that antidepressant therapy (and therapy with other psychoactive drugs) can be very helpful in selected terminally ill patients who suffer from severe depression.[33] The hospice/palliative care philosophy mandates attempts to relieve all types of suffering. For more information on the challenging task of assessing and managing nonphysical causes of pain and treating anxiety and depression, see *UNIPAC 2: Alleviating Psychological and Spiritual Pain in the Terminally Ill.*

Alleviating Intractable Terminal Suffering

While most patients experience excellent relief from suffering with the support of a hospice or palliative care team and the interventions outlined in this UNIPAC and others, some patients continue to suffer from intractable end-of-life problems. Sedation at the end of life (see UNIPACs 2, 6, and 8) and voluntary refusal of food and fluids are ethical and effective means of coping with intractable suffering, without resorting to assisted suicide.[34]

Effective treatment of pain depends on careful assessment, specific interventions designed to relieve each type of pain, and continuous reassessment of the patient's pain. When pain increases or remains uncontrolled, the practitioner should institute a thorough reassessment and consider the following:

- Disease progression versus treatable complications
- Need for increased dosages of opioids and/or adjuvant drugs
- Need for alternative routes of drug administration
- Presence of unresolved emotional and spiritual pain
- Problems with patient compliance or unacceptable side effects
- Need for increased involvement of other members of interdisciplinary team and medical specialists

Reassess for Total Pain

When reassessing for total pain, it is important to focus not only on new sources of physical pain caused by disease progression or other factors, but also on nonphysical causes of pain. Reassessment may reveal painful social, emotional, or spiritual issues that were missed during the initial assessment process, or new issues may have arisen that are causing distress for the patient and/or family. The physician should initiate a gentle and thorough investigation of all possible sources of the patient's suffering.

Reassess for Increased Involvement of Interdisciplinary Team

During the reassessment process, the physician should consider the need for increased involvement of hospice interdisciplinary team members and other healthcare professionals. Important issues to explore include these: Have members of the interdisciplinary team been adequately involved in caring for the patient and family? Have team members been providing effective interventions designed to relieve the suffering of this particular patient and family?[35] Do specific members of the team need to become more involved?

Members of the Interdisciplinary Team

- Chaplain
- Team physician
- Clinical psychologist
- Enterostomal therapist
- Home health aide
- Inpatient team
- Nurse
- Physical and/or occupational therapist
- Pharmacist
- Registered dietitian
- Social worker or counselor
- Hospice volunteer

Reassess Patient Compliance

Because patients and family members may be embarrassed to admit noncompliance, gentle but thorough and specific questioning is needed to determine levels of compliance. Is the patient complying with recommended treatments? Are concerns about opioid treatment interfering with regular dosing at prescribed levels? Is more patient and/or family education needed? Is the patient concerned about somnolence? Constipation? Is the patient skipping doses to ensure alertness?

Reassess Need for Increased Dosages of Opioids

Increase Dosages of Opioids

Is the current baseline dose still adequate to control pain? Is further titration necessary? Is a more potent opioid needed? Because no recommended dose exists that is adequate for every patient, opioids must be individually titrated to effectively control pain. With appropriate titration, no maximum ceiling dose exists. Some patients may require more than 2,000 mg of hydromorphone (Dilaudid) SC every day. However, such high doses can cause severe confusion, sedation, myoclonus, or even hyperalgesia. These side effects can be alleviated effectively by rotating to a less-than-equivalent dose of another potent opioid.

Consider Rotating to Methadone

Methadone has proved to be very effective for relieving severe pain in selected patients when high doses of other opioids are ineffective or result in unacceptable side effects.[36] Methadone can be administered PO, IV, PR, or SC (with dexamethasone or hyaluronidase).[37] The process of converting from other opioids to methadone is complex due to its long half-life. Conversion requires considerable attention, experience, and usually 3 to 6 days in an inpatient setting, where patients' highly variable reactions can be monitored closely.[38] The dose ratio of methadone to morphine or hydromorphone changes according to the total opioid dose. The common practice at the Palliative Care Unit in Edmonton, Canada is shown in Table 14.

Table 14: One Method of Rotating Opioids to Oral or Rectal Methadone

Day 1

- Decrease previous opioid dose by one-third.
- Replace with 3% of previous daily oral morphine equivalent dose, given as oral or rectal methadone every 8 h (e.g., a patient receiving 1,000 mg of oral morphine is switched to 660 mg of oral morphine + 30 mg per day of oral methadone, such as 10 mg PO or PR q 8 h).

Day 2

- Decrease previous opioid by another one-third **if** pain is controlled with rescue doses of a short-acting opioid.
- Increase methadone dose only if pain is moderate to severe.

Day 3

- Discontinue final one-third of previous opioid.
- For breakthrough pain, give patient a rescue dose of about 10% of the daily methadone dose, orally or rectally.
- Continue daily assessment of pain and dose titration until reaching an effective stable dose of methadone.

Adapted from Bruera E, Neumann CM. Role of methadone in the management of pain in cancer patients. *Oncology.* 1999;13(9):1275–82.

Reassess Need for Alternative Routes of Drug Administration

When pain continues despite the use of effective doses of oral morphine, other routes of drug administration should be investigated because:

- The patient may not be taking the prescribed oral morphine due to difficulties with swallowing.

- The absorption of oral morphine may be inhibited, e.g., in the case of delayed gastric emptying.

When ambulatory patients can no longer swallow, effective alternative routes for delivering medication include the following: sublingual, rectal, transdermal, and subcutaneous (or IV if a central venous catheter is in place). Intramuscular injections are rarely necessary.

Sublingual Administration

When patients are unable to swallow, immediate-release morphine or hydromorphone (Dilaudid) can be given sublingually. The soluble morphine tablets made by Eli Lilly and concentrated oral solutions (like Roxanol) are particularly effective for sublingual administration. Lipid-soluble opioids such as fentanyl are absorbed particularly well sublingually.

Rectal Administration

Opioids and many adjuvant medications are effectively absorbed from the rectum. Slow-release morphine tablets inserted into an empty, moist rectum can deliver 12 hours of analgesia, comparable to their effect when given orally.[39] Custom-made suppositories of methadone have proved effective at a wide range of doses.[38] A number of adjuvant analgesics, such as naproxen or valproic acid, can be administered rectally by instilling the oral solution into the rectum using an enema bulb, a urinary catheter, or a 6-inch length of nasal prongs oxygen tubing attached to a syringe. Some adjuvants, such as doxepin, come in gelatin capsules that dissolve in the rectum. Others can be crushed and put into large gel caps for insertion into the rectum.[29]

Transdermal Administration

Transdermal fentanyl patches (Duragesic) can deliver 3 days of effective, well-tolerated analgesia. The cost of using transdermal fentanyl patches is most clearly justified when

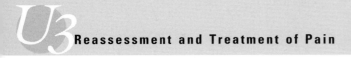

Table 15: Manufacturer's Suggested Starting Doses of Transdermal Fentanyl

Oral Morphine (mg/24 h)	Transdermal Fentanyl (mcg/h q 3 days)
45–134	25
135–224	50
225–314	75
315–404	100
405–494	125
495–584	150
585–674	175
675–764	200

NOTE: Do not use this table to convert from transdermal fentanyl to oral morphine. The doses of transdermal fentanyl are very conservative and will result in overestimation of the morphine dose.

patients cannot tolerate oral opioids. The effectiveness of transdermal fentanyl patches can be enhanced by:

- Prescribing a short-acting opioid for breakthrough pain during the first 24 hours, while the fentanyl reaches steady state
- Continuing the use of a short-acting opioid for breakthrough pain
- Close monitoring for dose titration

The table from the package insert (see Table 15) is very conservative. Up to 50% of patients will require dose titration to experience pain relief. For more robust patients, a simpler method of titration is often used: Divide the 24-hour total dose of oral morphine by 2 to get a starting dose of transdermal fentanyl.[40] For example, a patient taking 400 mg of oral morphine in 24 hours would be switched to 200 mcg/h transdermal fentanyl every 72 hours. Note the contrast between this regimen and the one recommended by the manufacturers in Table 15.

Do not use transdermal fentanyl or any other slow-release preparation when rapid dose titration is needed or when very accurate dosing is required (e.g., when a patient is beginning to experience respiratory failure or delirium). Use IV or SC boluses of shorter-acting opioids until the patient experiences relief, then use scheduled doses or a continuous infusion.

Subcutaneous Administration

Although the use of syringe drivers and other portable pumps is not yet common practice in all hospice programs in the United States, they offer a simple and effective means of pain control for many hospice patients without the pain or complications of IM or IV injections.[41] The technique is often initiated in an inpatient setting where the patient's response can be monitored carefully and the dose adjusted until optimal relief is achieved.

Patients who may benefit from continuous infusions include those with the following conditions:

- Persistent nausea and vomiting
- Severe dysphagia or swallowing disorders
- Delirium, confusion, or stupor
- High doses of oral medications that require numerous tablets

A simple syringe driver or other portable pump can deliver subcutaneous infusions of opioids, ketorolac, and some antiemetics through a small-gauge butterfly needle into the upper chest, outer arm, thigh, abdomen, or suprascapular region (see Figure 2).

Figure 2: Syringe Driver*

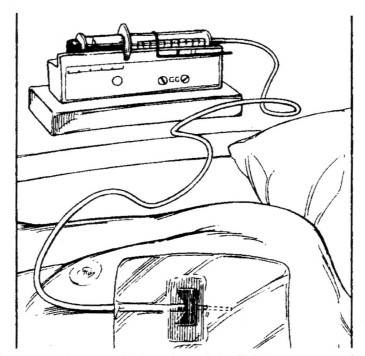

*The skin over the outer deltoid, suprascapular, or quadraceps is less likely to cause a pneumothorax than the pectoral area illustrated above.

The technique is safe, simple enough for home use, effective, and inexpensive. It allows for continued patient mobility if worn in a beltlike purse or shoulder holster. Subcutaneous infusion provides blood levels comparable to those from intravenous administration. Refer to the manual that accompanies the pump for appropriate settings.

Morphine and hydromorphone are the usual drugs of choice for continuous opioid infusions. Morphine can be used in dosage strengths up to 50 mg/mL, but due to its high solubility, hydromorphone is the usual drug of choice for high-dose infusions by the SC route.

- To calculate the required total daily dose of SC morphine, simply divide the patient's total daily requirement of oral morphine or equivalent by 3. For an hourly rate, divide the total daily dose of SC morphine by 24 (see Tables 2 and 3).

- To calculate the required total daily dose of SC hydromorphone, simply divide the total daily oral morphine dose by 20. For an hourly rate, divide the patient's total daily dose of SC hydromorphone by 24 (see Tables 2 and 3).

- Prescribe a booster dose for breakthrough pain or nausea. Usually 1 hour of medication every 15 minutes as needed is appropriate. If more than three or four boosts are needed in one 8-hour period, the baseline dose should be adjusted upward.

Example

- The patient was comfortable on 2 oxycodone with acetaminophen (Percocet) 5-mg tablets every 4 hours but now is too nauseated to tolerate PO medicines.

  5 mg of oxycodone (one tablet) = 7.5 mg of oral morphine

  15 mg oral morphine equivalent (2 tablets) × 6 doses/day = 90 mg/day

  90 mg oral morphine/day divided by 20 = 4.5 mg SC hydromorphone/day

- Observe the patient carefully when changing opioids. Due to limited cross-tolerance between opioids, some patients will require smaller doses when opioids are changed.

NOTE: Some patients may require as much as 500 to 2,000 mg per day of SC hydromorphone to control their pain, so concentrated hydromorphone solutions (50 to 200 mg/mL) may have to be mixed from powder.

Intravenous Administration

Intravenous (IV) administration is appropriate when the patient is already receiving IV therapy for other reasons or has a central venous catheter. The intravenous route provides the most rapid onset of analgesia, but the duration of relief after a bolus dose is shorter than with other routes. Continuous intravenous infusion provides a consistent level of analgesia and is used with a small pump, as with a subcutaneous infusion. Inserting central venous catheters or restarting peripheral IVs for opioid infusion is uncomfortable and unnecessary because the subcutaneous route is equally efficacious.

Topical or Transmucosal Application

Painful skin lesions can be treated effectively with a eutectic mixture of lidocaine and prilocaine (EMLA cream). The pain associated with open skin ulcers often can be alleviated by applying gauze soaked with morphine or morphine in hydrocolloid gel.[42]

Oral transmucosal fentanyl citrate (Actiq) has proved effective for breakthrough pain.[43] It is available in 200, 400, 600, 800, 1,200, and 1,600 mcg strengths. Although serum fentanyl levels exhibit dose-proportional pharmacokinetics,[44] the optimal dose cannot be predicted from the patient's around-the-clock opioid regimen; it must be determined by titration.[43]

Epidural or Intrathecal Administration

When the above methods do not provide acceptable relief, some carefully selected patients will benefit from a nerve block[46] or an epidural or intrathecal infusion of morphine or fentanyl, perhaps with bupivacaine or clonidine.[47]

Avoid Intramuscular (IM) Administration

This route is painful, inconvenient, and unnecessary because opioids are well absorbed subcutaneously.

Reassess Need for Adjuvant Drugs

Is an adjuvant drug needed to control pain that does not respond completely to opioid therapy? Are current doses of adjuvant drugs still adequate to control pain? Have new sources of nonopioid-responsive pain developed? Is a new class of drugs required? Should a new drug within the same class be tried? When adjuvant drugs are required, the correct dose of a potent opioid like oral morphine coupled with an effective adjuvant analgesic can provide effective relief from pain in over 90% of terminally ill patients. For severe pain unresponsive to the above measures, ketamine 0.1 to 0.2 mg/kg PO, IV, or SC has proved effective in a few patients.[48]

Reassess Need for Involvement of Other Medical Specialists

When pain persists, consider involving the following medical specialists:

- Radiation therapist
- Neurosurgeon
- Anesthesiologist
- Medical oncologist
- Orthopedist
- Psychiatrist

These medical specialists may be able to help control pain with procedures such as:

- Limited-course palliative radiation therapy
- Palliative chemotherapy
- Nerve blocks or spinal infusions
- Implantation of drug-infusion systems
- Bone stabilization
- Management of severe depression or delirium
- Neurosurgical ablation

Patients need not die with unrelieved pain, even in the rare cases when the pain management methods presented in this UNIPAC are not effective. When all else fails, continuous SC or IV administration of midazolam or barbiturates can provide relaxed unconsciousness during the final days of life.[49]

The Assessment and Management of Pain

William and Evelyn G.

William G. is a 63-year-old male veteran who was diagnosed 1 year ago with adenocarcinoma of the lung, metastatic to the other lung. He has undergone radiation therapy and one dose of chemotherapy that caused such severe nausea and vomiting that he refused further treatment. He was referred for hospice care.

During the hospice physician's home assessment visit in William and Evelyn's modest home, William complains of severe pain that does not respond to the oral 4 mg hydromorphone (Dilaudid) tablets prescribed by his attending physician every 4 hours as needed for pain. During the interview William moans and reports all-over, aching pain, but is unable to rate it on a numerical scale. He is obviously miserable.

Question One

What is the most appropriate course of action to take now?

A. Prescribe a higher dose of hydromorphone (Dilaudid).

B. Add an adjuvant drug.

C. Order a set of electrolytes and blood urea nitrogen.

D. Transfer William to the hospital for IV morphine.

E. Perform a complete history and physical.

Correct Response and Analysis

The correct response is E. A thorough history and physical are required to adequately assess multiple causes of pain. In this case, more information is needed about the causes of William's pain before any decisions are made about medication orders or tests. The simple maneuver of completing a history and physical is much more likely to be productive and will cause the patient the least amount of pain and expense. Blood chemistries and counts will not provide the essential information needed.

The Case Continues: History and Physical Exam

The physician's first questions relate to the location of William's pain. When asked to point to all the places where he hurts, William eventually indicates his chest, stomach, and back. William clearly has tenderness on his chest wall and sacrum and is experiencing cramping discomfort in the lower abdomen.

The history further reveals that William is bed bound most of the time and needs assistance with turning. When discussing his medication, William says that he had been taking acetaminophen with codeine but it did not control the pain, so his physician prescribed hydromorphone (Dilaudid). He reports falling asleep after taking 4 mg of hydromorphone (Dilaudid) and then feeling somewhat drowsy and confused when he awakens. Although he is experiencing persistent pain, he takes only 1 hydromorphone (Dilaudid) tablet every other day because he wants to remain awake. The history also reveals that William has not had a bowel movement in 4 days. His wife is arthritic and is having increasing difficulty caring for William.

The physical exam reveals a cachectic male who appears older than his stated age. The exam is remarkable for decreased breath sounds on both sides of his chest, tenderness to the left side of the chest wall near the radiation therapy skin changes, and mild lower abdominal distention consistent with constipation. The rectal exam reveals a soft fecal impaction but no masses. He has a Stage II decubitus on his sacrum and severe muscle wasting.

Question Two

The four most likely causes of William's pain are:

A. Neuropathic pain

B. Bony and soft tissue pain from lung cancer

C. Pain from a decubitus ulcer

D. Pain from constipation

E. Underutilization of pain medication

Correct Response and Analysis

The correct responses are B, C, D, and E. William describes his pain as "all over and aching" and has chest-wall tenderness underneath the radiation therapy marks, both of which indicate the presence of bone and soft tissue pain resulting from bone and tissue involvement. William has a bedsore consistent with decreased mobility and lack of turning, he describes lower abdominal cramping consistent with not having had a bowel movement in 4 days, and he is noncompliant with analgesia orders because the hydromorphone (Di-

laudid) causes drowsiness and he wants to stay awake.

A is incorrect. Neuropathic pain appears to be an unlikely source of pain because the patient does not describe the stinging, burning, radiating pain along nerve distribution routes that usually characterizes such pain.

The Case Continues: Nonphysical Causes of Pain

Further discussion with William reveals that he is extremely angry and depressed about being fired from his job immediately after being diagnosed with cancer. He is worried that the financial pressures created by his illness will result in the loss of their home, leaving his wife with no place to live. Evelyn is fearful about how she is going to manage now that William can no longer provide financial support.

Question Three

Based on current information, which two of the following are the most likely causes of William's nonphysical pain?

A. Emotional or psychological pain

B. Social pain

C. Spiritual pain

Correct Response and Analysis

The correct responses are A and B. In this situation William expresses emotional pain, evidenced by his anger and depression, and social pain as evidenced by his worry about financial matters. Although William is likely to also be experiencing spiritual pain, he has not yet voiced such concerns.

Question Four

How might William's social and emotional pain affect the course of his illness?

A. They are irrelevant to the management of William's care.

B. They are likely to complicate medication compliance.

C. They are likely to exacerbate physical pain.

D. They are likely to impede William's acceptance of his approaching death.

Correct Response and Analysis

The correct answers are B, C, and D. Concerns about the cost of purchasing medicines may interfere with William's compliance with medication orders. Both emotional and social pain create stress and anxiety that can exacerbate physical pain and interfere with the acceptance of approaching death. William is unlikely to rest comfortably until his financial problems are addressed.

The Case Continues

During the first visit to William and Evelyn's home, the physician further explores William's reasons for not taking the hydromorphone (Dilaudid) as prescribed and discovers:

- William is concerned about drug addiction and says drowsiness and confusion are unacceptable side effects for him.

- Evelyn also is afraid of drug addiction and has been hiding the hydromorphone (Dilaudid). She wants William to stay awake so that he will eat more and regain his strength.

The physician determines that patient and family education is needed and explains the following:

- Taking pain medications for cancer pain does not lead to addiction; William can gradually stop taking his medication if his pain goes away completely.

- The drowsiness and confusion are occurring because he isn't taking medication of the appropriate strength.

- A different medication can be used that won't be quite as strong and won't cause as much drowsiness and confusion.

- It will be necessary to take the new medication on a regularly scheduled, 4-hour basis.

- Mild drowsiness may occur for the first day or two, but it won't be as bothersome as it has been with the hydromorphone (Dilaudid), and William's body will adjust to the new medicine after a day or two.

- William will be more awake and able to eat and won't be in as much pain.

- Evelyn should call the hospice if William becomes so sleepy that he can't be aroused to take his next dose of medicine; the dose will be reduced.

- William should take a booster dose if pain occurs, but should call the hospice if he has to take booster doses more than 2 or 3 times in a 24-hour period so that the baseline dose can be increased.

- The dose of the new medication will probably have to be adjusted up or down in the next few days, depending on how it works for William.

- Evelyn can call the hospice any time, day or night, if she has concerns about William's condition.

■ All of them are working together to relieve William's pain.

William and Evelyn agree that mild drowsiness for a day or two is an acceptable side effect. To determine the right starting dose of a new medication, the physician:

■ Calculates that William's 4 mg dose of hydromorphone (Dilaudid) is roughly equivalent to 20 mg of an oral morphine (oral hydromorphone is about five times as potent as oral morphine). See Table 2.

■ Decides that 20 mg of oral morphine equivalent is more than William needs to control his pain, but that 1–2 mg is not adequate because the Tylenol 3 that William had been taking prior to the hydromorphone (Dilaudid) did not provide relief.

■ Concludes that 7.5 mg of an oral morphine equivalent every 4 hours is a good place to start because William is a normal-sized adult weighing more than 60 pounds with severe pain and it is important to avoid unacceptable side effects.

Question Five

At this point, which of the following medications is an appropriate choice?

A. Oxycodone and acetaminophen (Percocet) 1 tablet every 4 hours, or

B. Acetaminophen 1,000 mg every 4 hours (alone), or

C. Slow-release morphine 60 mg every 12 hours, or

D. Slow-release morphine 15 mg three times daily, or

E. Transdermal fentanyl patches (Duragesic) one 50 mcg per hour patch every 72 hours

Correct Response and Analysis

Correct answers are A or D. The preferable response is (A) oxycodone and acetaminophen (Percocet) because:

■ Oxycodone 5 mg with acetaminophen (Percocet) is a cost-effective and widely available medication in this potency range (7.5 mg of oral morphine equivalent).

■ An immediate-release preparation allows more flexibility when rapid-dose titration is needed to establish an effective baseline dose.

■ In addition to his regular 4-hour dose, William needs medication for breakthrough pain. By prescribing oxycodone and acetaminophen (Percocet), one medication can be used for both purposes.

■ The presence of acetaminophen may be helpful, and William has no contraindicating symptoms; however, the acetaminophen limits the number of tablets that can be taken.

■ Evelyn is available to administer the oxycodone and acetaminophen (Percocet) every 4 hours.

■ Oxycodone without acetaminophen might be as effective and can be prescribed in higher doses, but is not as widely available.

The second-choice response is (D) slow-release morphine 15 mg three times daily because:

- It is roughly equivalent to 7.5 mg of oral morphine every 4 hours.

- It is about the same dose as the oxycodone and acetaminophen (Percocet), but does not provide the added benefit of acetaminophen.

- Two medications are necessary: slow-release morphine for the baseline dose and immediate release morphine for breakthrough pain. Using the fewest possible number of drugs is a goal of all medicine, in particular hospice medicine.

The Case Continues

The physician explains that (1) William must take one tablet every 4 hours around the clock, (2) he can take 1/2 tablet for breakthrough pain, and (3) at bedtime he can take 2 tablets so that he doesn't have to set an alarm clock to take his 2 AM dose. The physician then writes out a chart so that William and Evelyn can check when he has taken his tablet at 6 AM, 10 AM, 2 PM, 6 PM, and 2 tablets at 10 PM.

Laxative Regimen

The physician does the following: (1) orders bisacodyl (Dulcolax) suppositories, (2) suggests that William insert one suppository as soon as possible, (3) explains that the medication usually works within an hour, (4) recommends using 2 suppositories if the first one is ineffective, (5) encourages the use of a suppository if a bowel movement does not occur at least every other day, and (6) asks Evelyn to call the hospice if William needs to use the suppositories regularly. The physician also prescribes Senokot S (senna with docusate), 1 tablet twice daily, to prevent recurrent constipation.

Team Involvement

The physician concludes the visit by making arrangements for the hospice nurse and social worker to visit with William and Evelyn the next day to (1) make sure that William is comfortable and awake, (2) reinforce what the physician has said about addiction, and (3) explore the family's financial needs and help them to obtain available community assistance.

Evelyn calls the hospice at midnight the next night and reports that William is experiencing a lot of chest pain. The hospice RN confirms that (1) William has been taking one tablet of oxycodone and acetaminophen (Percocet) every 4 hours, (2) that his bowel movements are occurring regularly, and (3) that the pain has the same character and location as before, and so it is most likely chest wall pain from the lung cancer.

Question Six

At this point, which of the following is an appropriate order?

A. Morphine solution (morphine 20 mg/mL) 1 cc every 4 hours

B. Oxycodone and acetaminophen 2 tablets every 4 hours

C. Hydromorphone 4 mg every 4 hours

D. Slow-release morphine 15 mg every 12 hours

Correct Response and Analysis

Correct responses are either B or D. Both are equivalent to 10 mg of oral morphine, but (B) oxycodone and acetaminophen is the preferred response because, as the titration process continues, an immediate-release product allows more flexibility in dosing. However, at midnight it will be difficult to locate a new opioid, so a higher dose of whichever drug was selected in Question Five is the best answer.

Responses A and C are incorrect because the suggested doses are too strong.

The Case Continues

The hospice RN increases the oxycodone and acetaminophen to 2 tablets every 4 hours with a whole tablet for breakthrough pain. William is comfortable by morning.

A few days later, William is at home in a hospital bed and has an alternating pressure pad for his decubitus. Evelyn has been taught how to reposition him on a regular basis. The social worker has arranged for the following: (1) the utility company will waive William and Evelyn's overdue payments, (2) the Veterans Administration hospital will provide medications, and (3) procedures for obtaining disability payments have been initiated. The hospice chaplain has arranged for regular visits from William and Evelyn's pastor at their request.

On the next visit 3 days later, the nurse discovers that William is getting good pain relief with 2 oxycodone and acetaminophen tablets, but is sometimes confused and occasionally sees people on the wall. Evelyn thinks William is overmedicated.

Question Seven

At this point, what is the best choice for a medication order?

A. Add aspirin 325 mg every 4 hours.

B. Order an epidural catheter.

C. Reduce oxycodone and acetaminophen (Percocet) and add naproxen (Naprosyn).

D. Order an IV infusion pump.

E. Add amitriptyline at bedtime.

Correct Response and Analysis

William obtains good pain relief with 2 oxycodone and acetaminophen tablets, but the side effects are unacceptable. At this point the physician has two available options: (1) choose a different opioid in an attempt to reduce side effects or (2) lower the analgesia dose to decrease side effects and add an adjuvant to enhance analgesia.

The best response is C, reduce the oxycodone and acetaminophen to 1 tablet every 4 hours to relieve side effects and add naproxen (Naprosyn) 375 mg twice daily to control chest wall pain.

This situation illustrates the correct use of co-analgesics. When patients experience bone pain, it is not always necessary to immediately begin treatment with a co-analgesic such as naproxen (Naprosyn). Because such drugs are more toxic than morphine or oxycodone and acetaminophen, it is appropriate to begin treatment with morphine or oxycodone and acetaminophen and add naproxen (Naprosyn) only when needed.

(A) is an incorrect response. Aspirin 325 mg every 4 hours would help to relieve chest wall pain, but is much more toxic to the stomach lining than naproxen (Naprosyn) and would not alleviate the opioid side effects. (B) is an incorrect response. An epidural catheter is invasive and expensive, and simpler maneuvers such as adding a different adjuvant have not been tried. (D) ordering an IV infusion pump is incorrect for the same reason as (B). (E) is incorrect because amitriptyline may increase William's confusion.

The Case Concludes

The next day the RN reports that William's pain is moderately well controlled, but he is taking extra doses three times a day. The physician increases the naproxen (Naprosyn) to 375 mg three times a day with good relief of chest wall pain and no return of the confusion.

After several weeks William's pain begins to increase, so he is switched to oral morphine 15 mg every 4 hours with good pain control and no additional side effects. William eventually becomes weaker, is more confused, and has difficulty swallowing. He appears to be approaching death. The hospice team elects to switch William to morphine soluble tablets 20 mg every 4 hours, which Evelyn dissolves in a few drops of water and puts just inside William's lip. Indomethacin suppositories, 50 mg every 4 hours for antiinflammatory effects, are added. This regimen keeps William comfortable until he dies, at which time the hospice program initiates bereavement care for Evelyn.

Mildred T.

Mildred T. is a widow with multiple myeloma who lives in a nursing home. Despite several courses of melphalan (Alkeran) and prednisone, she complains of severe, all-over, deep pain. The nursing home staff reports that Mildred complains a lot, has intermittent periods of confusion, and is more depressed, irritable, and withdrawn than before. Her present medications are hydrocodone with acetaminophen 5/500 mg (Vicodin) 1 tablet q 4 hours as needed for pain; levothyroxin 0.1 mg per day; milk of magnesia 30 cc as needed for constipation; docusate (Colace), and a multiple vitamin.

Remembering what you have learned from this UNIPAC, you complete a careful history and physical. Among other problems, the history reveals that Mildred has right hip pain on weight bearing that eases at rest. She also has left-sided chest wall pain, particularly when she leans forward. She has been taking approximately 2 hydrocodone with acetaminophen (Vicodin) tablets per day and has had a soft bowel movement every other day. She has not taken milk of magnesia in more than a week. During the interview, Mildred is grumpy and withdrawn. She rates her pain as an 8 on a 10-point scale.

The physical exam reveals a very neatly dressed 68-year-old female who has just tried to arrange her snow-white hair. Mildred is of short stature with a small distance between her iliac crest and lower rib cage, suggestive of vertebral compression fractures. Her abdomen is somewhat protuberant, but she is not obese. Her extremities show some muscle wasting and trace edema in her ankles. Her legs are of equal length, and she can move all her joints passively without discomfort. Her chest is clear, but she winces when the stethoscope is placed on the left side of her rib cage. Her skin is in good condition.

Question One

The two most likely causes of Mildred's pain are:

A. Visceral cramping

B. Neuropathic pain

C. Bone and soft tissue pain due to rib involvement

D. Constipation

E. Bone pain due to right hip involvement

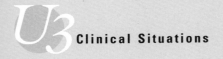

Correct Response and Analysis

The correct answers are C and E. Mildred is receiving inadequate analgesic relief from the hydrocodone with acetaminophen (Vicodin), which may be due to the fact that she is not taking it on a regular around-the-clock schedule. Her aching all-over pain, coupled with rib cage tenderness, is consistent with bone and soft tissue pain due to rib involvement. The hip pain that increases on weight bearing but eases at rest is consistent with bone pain resulting from hip involvement. Mildred has had soft bowel movements every other day, and her pain does not seem to be abdominal.

The Case Continues: Additional Information from History

Further discussion with Mildred reveals that she is furious with her daughter for putting her in a nursing home and is depressed about losing her lifelong home and belongings. She particularly mourns the loss of weekly visits to her hairdresser, shopping at the mall with her friends, and the lovely clothes that she used to wear. Mildred is angry with the nursing staff and now believes that she is not receiving adequate care in the nursing home. Her sleep is disturbed and she refuses to swallow her medications until her pain becomes unbearable, but she will not discuss her reasons for refusing. She will not consent to an evaluation for palliative radiotherapy.

Question Two

At this time Mildred is experiencing physical, emotional, and social pain. Choose the four most likely effects of the nonphysical components of her pain.

A. They will affect medication compliance.

B. They are likely to worsen and should be reported to the hospice social worker and counseling staff.

C. They will exacerbate her physical pain.

D. They will make her less likely to tolerate medication side effects.

E. They are untreatable and will result in the need for psychiatric consultations.

Correct Response and Analysis

The correct responses are A, B, C, and D. Mildred's anger at her daughter appears to be affecting her relationship with the nursing facility staff. Both her refusal to discuss her noncompliance with medication orders and the severity of her nonphysical pain suggest the presence of complicated psychosocial issues that should be addressed by all members of the hospice team, including a social worker or other counselor. Mildred's anger and probable depression and anxiety will cause not only emotional pain, but will also exacerbate her physical pain and her ability to tolerate medication side effects. They will also affect her judgment when she considers treatment options such as palliative radiation.

Review Question Three

At this time, which one of the following medications is the most appropriate choice to control Mildred's pain?

A. Hydromorphone (Dilaudid) 2 mg PO every 4 hours

B. Slow-release morphine 30 mg PO twice daily

C. Transdermal fentanyl patches (Duragesic) 50 mcg/h 1 patch q 2 to 3 days

D. Hydrocodone with acetaminophen 1 tablet PO every 4 hours

E. Amitriptyline (Elavil) 50 mg PO at bedtime

Correct Response and Analysis

The correct answer is D. Hydrocodone with acetaminophen (Vicodin) 1 tablet every 4 hours is a good initial choice. Instead of switching to a more potent medication, the most appropriate action at this time is to increase the dosing frequency of the medication that she is currently taking from 2 tablets a day to 1 tablet every 4 hours. The medication is not causing unacceptable side effects, and she has no complaints of drowsiness, hallucinations, or itching. Constipation, a common side effect, has been addressed with a laxative.

Reminders: Hydrocodone with acetaminophen 5 mg is roughly equivalent to 2 mg of oral morphine; an accompanying order should be written for extra doses for breakthrough pain—in this case, an appropriate order would be 1/2 tablet of hydrocodone with acetaminophen every 2 hours as needed when Mildred complains of pain.

Choices A, B, C, and E are incorrect. Two milligrams of hydromorphone (Dilaudid) every 4 hours is equivalent to 8 mg of oral morphine, which is four times as potent as the hydrocodone with acetaminophen. In this case, such a dramatic increase in drug potency is not indicated and would probably cause unacceptable side effects.

Slow-release morphine 30 mg and transdermal fentanyl patches (Duragesic) are inappropriate for the same reasons. Although it provides smooth, continuous pain relief, slow-release morphine 30 mg every 12 hours is equivalent to 10 mg of oral morphine every 4 hours, a dose that is 5 times as potent as the hydrocodone with acetaminophen and is likely to cause unacceptable side effects. The 50-mcg transdermal fentanyl patch (Duragesic) is equivalent to 11 to 18 mg of oral morphine every 4 hours, which is 5 to 9 times as potent as hydrocodone with acetaminophen. Once again, a dramatic increase in potency is not indicated and is likely to create unacceptable side effects. Amitriptyline is incorrect. Although amitriptyline can be a useful addition to an opioid analgesia regimen when treating neuropathic pain, this type of pain is not a factor in this case, and amitriptyline by itself is unlikely to provide adequate analgesia.

The Case Continues

In this case, as in most others, multiple interventions are required. The physician gently explores several issues with Mildred, including her reasons for not taking the medication on a regular basis and her anger with her daughter and the nursing home staff. Further discussion reveals that Mildred objects to taking the hydrocodone with acetaminophen every 4 hours because she has known people who "got hooked" on tranquilizers, and she doesn't want to become a drug addict. She thinks her daughter wants to "dope her up" so she won't complain.

The physician carefully explains the difference between physical dependence and psychological addiction, quotes medical literature about the extreme rarity of psychological addiction in cancer patients,[12] explains that the hydrocodone with acetaminophen is simply counteracting the effects of the multiple myeloma, and stresses the importance of taking 1 hydrocodone with acetaminophen on a regular 4-hour schedule. After Mildred is assured that she will be able to stop taking hydrocodone with acetaminophen with no problems if her pain goes away, she agrees to the 4-hour schedule.

Orders are written for 1 hydrocodone with acetaminophen tablet every 4 hours on a regular basis, except at bedtime, when 2 tablets are prescribed so that Mildred can skip the 2 AM dose and sleep through the night. The only likely side effect of the double dose at bedtime is increased sedation, which is desirable at night.

After switching to the new regime, Mildred discovers that her pain is adequately controlled at rest, but she continues to experience severe pain in her hip when she tries to get out of bed and walk. Additional doses before getting out of bed do not control the pain on walking. The nurse and social worker report that Mildred's depressive symptoms have begun to improve following the relief of pain and talks with the hospice counselor.

Better pain control and counseling help to alleviate interpersonal problems that appeared deeply rooted and resistant to intervention. With the help of the hospice counselor, Mildred is able to reflect on several issues, including her long-term relationship with her daughter, her daughter's fight for independence, and her own feelings of rejection. As Mildred's psychosocial and physical pain are controlled, her suffering decreases.

Review Question Four

Which one of the following is the best choice for controlling Mildred's pain on movement?

A. Transdermal fentanyl patches (Duragesic) 50 mcg per hour 1 patch q 3 days

B. Physical therapy for progressive ambulation exercises

C. Oxycodone and acetaminophen 1 to 2 tablets every 4 hours plus ibuprofen 400 mg every 4 hours

D. Amitriptyline at bedtime in addition to the hydrocodone with acetaminophen

E. Slow-release morphine 30 mg every 8 hours

Correct Response and Analysis

The correct answer is C. Pain that occurs only on movement can be difficult to control because the amount of analgesic necessary to control pain on movement may be too much at rest. Because Mildred is comfortable at rest, a dramatic increase in dose is likely to cause increased side effects. Oxycodone and acetaminophen offer a moderate increase in potency, and ibuprofen is an appropriate adjuvant drug for bone and soft tissue pain that may add additional analgesia without compromising her mental status.

If pain persists despite the use of ibuprofen, a brief course of palliative radiation therapy may relieve Mildred's pain if she has not already received radiation to that area and agrees to the treatment. Transdermal fentanyl patches (Duragesic) and slow-release morphine are incorrect. Even though the increased opioid dose might be helpful when she is up and moving, the same dose is likely to cause excessive drowsiness and confusion while at rest. Amitriptyline is incorrect. As an adjuvant, amitriptyline is much more likely to help to relieve neuropathic pain than bone and soft tissue pain. In this case, neuropathic pain is not an issue, and Mildred's depressive symptoms are already resolving.

The Case Continues

When the physician visits the nursing home again, Mildred is using her walker to walk down the hall. She is grateful for the physician's efforts to control her pain, but says she doesn't have time to talk because a bridge game is starting in a few minutes. Mildred mentions mild discomfort on movement, but says it is not enough to keep her immobile. She doesn't want to bother with radiation therapy.

Mildred enjoys 6 weeks of good pain control during which time her strength gradually declines. Her ibuprofen is decreased and misoprostol added due to stomach upset, but otherwise her symptoms remain under good control.

One day Mildred develops a temperature, becomes too weak to get out of bed, has difficulty swallowing her ibuprofen and oxycodone and acetaminophen tablets, and is unable to respond with more than one syllable when the nurse asks her a question. The physician examines her and suspects pneumonia or a urinary tract infection and discusses the situation with Mildred and her daughter. A decision is made to withhold antibiotic treatment because Mildred's condition appears to be part of the natural course of her myeloma, and she has always insisted that she does not want the debilitating stage of her disease to be prolonged.

Mildred has been taking 2 oxycodone and acetaminophen tablets every 4 hours and 400-mg ibuprofen every 8 hours, but is now unable to swallow such large pills.

Review Question Five

Which of the following will provide pain relief in a simple but effective manner?

A. Slow-release morphine 30 tablet mg every 8 hours PO or per rectum

B. Transdermal fentanyl patch (Duragesic) 50 μg per hour 1 patch every 3 days with Indocin 50 mg q 12 hours per rectum

C. IV morphine at 5 mg per hour

D. PCA pump delivering hydromorphone (Dilaudid) at 0.5 mg per hour (basal rate) with 0.5 mg q 30 minutes prn (PCA)

E. Transfer to hospital for further evaluation

Correct Response and Analysis

The best responses are either A or B. The transdermal fentanyl patch (Duragesic) provides an oral morphine equivalent of about 16 mg every 4 hours, which is less than a 50% increase over the oxycodone and acetaminophen, is noninvasive, does not require the ability to swallow tablets, and is much easier to manage than an IV or PCA pump in a nursing home situation. Slow-release morphine (MS Contin and probably Oramorph SR) tablets are absorbed rectally about as well as by mouth. In either case, sublingual morphine 5 mg as needed would be an adequate booster dose.

Incorrect responses are C, D, and E. A continuous IV infusion of morphine at 5 mg per hour is the equivalent of 60 mg of oral morphine every 4 hours, a dose that is much too potent and is likely to cause confusion and could result in Mildred's attempting to pull out the peripheral line. This route is also difficult to manage in a nursing home.

A PCA pump also requires a peripheral IV unless it is delivered subcutaneously, but requiring Mildred to punch a button to control pain is neither

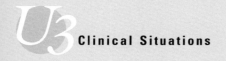
realistic nor appropriate given her fever and decreasing mental status.

A transfer is unnecessary because Mildred's symptoms can be adequately controlled in the nursing home. In addition, a decision has been made to forgo aggressive treatment of the complications of her myeloma, so there is no need for acute care. Mildred does not want the debilitating stage of her illness to be prolonged, and she might get less pain relief in a hospital.

The Case Concludes

Using these measures, Mildred is able to remain in the nursing home in relative comfort. She develops rattling secretions that are controlled with 2 scopolamine patches (Transderm Scop) and dies comfortably 2 days later in the presence of her daughter. Mildred's daughter and the nursing home staff are grateful for the hospice/palliative care interventions.

NOTE: Although the tendency among many physicians is to classify every psychosocial problem as a mental health issue and immediately write a prescription for a psychoactive drug or make a psychiatric referral, other actions may be more appropriate. Before prescribing medication to relieve mild to moderate anxiety and depression, the practitioner should first attempt nondrug measures, such as facilitating good communication that includes careful listening and brief counseling. During the communication process, physicians should be sensitive to the severity of the patient's psychosocial or spiritual problems and to their own levels of competence, and, when necessary, refer the patient to other members of the interdisciplinary team or to an outside specialist.

Physicians and patients vary in their willingness to talk about psychosocial and spiritual issues. When patients and their physicians want to dis-

cuss such issues, the physician should schedule enough time to sit down and thoroughly explore troubling issues. When physicians are uncomfortable talking about spiritual or psychological issues, patients should be referred to other members of the interdisciplinary team, such as the social worker, counselor, chaplain, or volunteer. However, in this case the physician's initial assessment may be a valuable addition to assessments made by other team members. By working together, health care professionals are more likely to offer effective interventions that relieve not just physical pain, but also the pain caused by spiritual and psychosocial issues.

Dennis and Jean D., a Test Clinical Situation

(See the correct responses at the end of this clinical situation.)

Dennis D. is a male dentist with carcinoma of the stomach who has just been referred for hospice/palliative care. He has had several courses of chemotherapy, none of which slowed the progression of his disease. He is taking the following medications: 30 mg of slow-release morphine twice a day, 25 mg of chlorpromazine (Thorazine) three times a day for nausea, 50 mg of amitriptyline (Elavil) at bedtime for sleep, and 2 senna 5 mg plus docusate 100 mg (Senokot S) tablets twice daily for constipation.

During the physician's assessment visit to Dennis and Jean's beautifully appointed home, Dennis complains of abdominal pain that he describes as 7.2 overall on a 10-point scale. He says the pain sometimes feels cramping and fluctuates from a 3 to a 9 depending on whether or not he has just urinated.

Remembering what you have learned from this UNIPAC, you complete a careful history and physical. The history reveals a man who needs to urinate almost hourly throughout the day and night and requires his wife's assistance to walk from their bed to the bathroom. Both Dennis and Jean are exhausted from interrupted sleep and the physical difficulty of making such frequent trips to the bathroom. Dennis has had a moderate-sized bowel movement each day during the past 7 days.

The physical exam reveals a bald, 42-year-old male with a clear chest, an abdomen that is tender in the upper quadrants with a rock-hard mass in the epigastric area, and a large round mass just above the pubis. His extremities show muscle wasting and trace edema.

Question One

Three likely causes of Dennis's lower abdominal pain are:

A. Tumor involvement of viscera

B. Ureteral obstruction by tumor

C. Urinary retention

D. Poor medication compliance

E. Medication side effects

NOTE: Consider the combined anticholinergic effects of morphine, chlorpromazine (Thorazine), and amitriptyline (Elavil).

The Case Continues: Additional Information from History

Further discussion reveals that Dennis is anguished about leaving his two young children without a father and is very concerned about his rapidly decreasing ability to function physically. When Jean leaves the room, the physician asks if anything else is troubling him and Dennis begins to weep quietly.

He reveals a troubled marriage that was further threatened by an affair he had just before he became ill. Dennis has been active in his church and questions whether his illness is a punishment for his affair. He is overwhelmed with guilt and hates having to constantly rely on his wife.

Question Two

Which three of the following types of non-physical pain appear to be causing distress in this case?

A. Emotional pain

B. Neuropathic pain

C. Social pain

D. Spiritual pain

E. Financial pain

Question Three

Which three responses best describe how nonphysical pain is likely to affect the course of Dennis's illness?

A. It is irrelevant to the treatment and management of this case.

B. It is likely to affect Dennis's acceptance of the catheter he may need to relieve his urinary retention.

C. It is unlikely he will be able to tolerate the withdrawal of the chlorpromazine and amitriptyline that are causing his urinary retention unless other medications are prescribed to treat his anxiety and depression.

D. It is likely to greatly exacerbate his suffering regardless of medication.

E. A psychiatric referral will be necessary.

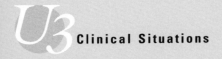

The Case Continues

The chlorpromazine (Thorazine) and amitriptyline (Elavil) are discontinued, and haloperidol (Haldol) 1 mg twice daily is substituted for control of nausea, with lorazepam 1 mg at bedtime to help with sleep. Dennis's urinary retention subsides, but he still complains of moderate amounts of upper abdominal pain. The physician and nurse agree that this pain seems to be the result of tumor involvement of his stomach, so the physician increases the slow-release morphine to 30 mg three times a day. *Note:* Slow release morphine tablets usually last 12 hours, but may be prescribed every 8 hours to evenly distribute 90 mg of morphine over 24 hours.

The increased dose of slow-release morphine helps temporarily, but causes unacceptable amounts of drowsiness. Without consulting the physician, Dennis reduces his slow-release morphine dose to 30 mg twice daily with the return of unacceptable levels of pain.

E. Start a morphine drip at 2 mg per hour, with 1 mg every 30 minutes if needed.

The Case Continues

The physician asks Dennis to try the new medication, but warns him that a change in medication might cause drowsiness for a day or two. Dennis reluctantly agrees, and 3 days later his wife reports that Dennis is mentally clear, much more comfortable, and able to urinate. With the help of the hospice chaplain, Dennis and Jean make progress with giving and receiving forgiveness, which further increases his comfort. However, as the weeks pass, Dennis's strength continues to deteriorate, and he becomes bedbound and intermittently confused. The pain in his abdomen begins to require frequent extra doses of the new medication, and one night his wife has to give him additional doses every 2 hours throughout the night. He is having great difficulty swallowing tablets.

Question Four

Which one of the following is the best course of action to relieve Dennis's pain?

A. Continue the slow-release morphine with instructions that Dennis must take it if he wants good pain relief.

B. Give 15 mg of immediate-release morphine every 4 hours with 10-mg morphine every 2 hours if needed for breakthrough pain.

C. Add doxepin (Sinequan) 50 mg at bedtime.

D. Switch from morphine to hydromorphone (Dilaudid) 4 mg every 4 hours with 2-mg hydromorphone every 2 hours if needed.

Question Five

At this time, which one of the following is the most appropriate (effective and least invasive) course of action?

A. Transfer Dennis to the hospital for a celiac plexus block.

B. Insert an epidural catheter for epidural morphine infusion.

C. Begin an SC infusion of hydromorphone (Dilaudid) at 8 mg per day.

D. Begin a PCA pump with hydromorphone (Dilaudid) at 1 mg every 15 minutes as needed.

E. Tell Jean that Dennis's confusion is expected and she should carry on as before.

The Case Continues

Jean calls the next day to report that Dennis's pain is well controlled and that both of them were able to sleep. Several days later, she calls again to report that Dennis has become restless and agitated and is calling out to people who are not there. Jean is very distressed by this new symptom. All efforts to talk with Dennis about what is going on are unsuccessful because he is unable to concentrate on the questions.

Question Six

Which of the following interventions would be appropriate at this time?

A. Double the infusion dose of hydromorphone (Dilaudid).

B. Add haloperidol (Haldol) 5 mg per day and midazolam (Versed) 5 mg per day to the hydromorphone (Dilaudid) infusion **or** use chlorpromazine (Thorazine) 25- to 50-mg suppositories per rectum q 4-6 hours as needed.

C. Transfer Dennis to a hospice inpatient unit for intensive symptom control.

D. Discontinue the opioid analgesic.

E. Order secobarbital (Seconal) 100 mg tablets #50 and let Jean know that Dennis will die if she gives all of them to him.

The Case Concludes

Dennis dies 2 days later from natural causes, and

Jean is grateful for the hospice/palliative care interventions.

Test Clinical Situation Correct Responses

1. A, C, and E are correct because Dennis has a rock-hard mass consistent with tumor involvement of the viscera that is likely to be causing pain, and the combined anticholinergic side effects of morphine, chlorpromazine (Thorazine), and amitriptyline (Elavil) are likely to be causing urinary retention. B and D are incorrect because Dennis's bladder contains urine and he is complying with the medication orders.

2. A, C, and D are the most appropriate responses because Dennis has voiced feelings of guilt, anguish about leaving two small children, and concerns about being punished for his behavior. B is incorrect because neuropathic pain is not a nonphysical cause of pain and because Dennis does not describe his pain as burning, shooting, or stabbing. E is less likely to be correct than the other responses because Dennis has not yet voiced any financial concerns and he appears to have adequate financial resources.

3. B is correct because a catheter may be viewed by Dennis as one more sign of his increasing dependence or as a symbol of punishment for his affair. C and D are correct because Dennis is likely to need medication to treat anxiety and depression and because nonphysical pain contributes to total pain and exacerbates suffering. Response A is incorrect because the components of total pain are interactive; Dennis' emotional, spiritual, and social pain are likely to exacerbate his physical pain. E is incorrect because Dennis' nonphysical

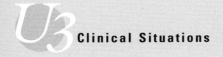

causes of pain can likely be alleviated with effective symptom control and support from the hospice team.

4. D is correct because rotating opioids may reduce unacceptable side effects. Response A is incorrect because attempts should be made to alleviate distressing side effects. B, C, and E are incorrect because they are unlikely to reduce drowsiness. The opioid doses are higher than was acceptable to Dennis, and doxepin can be very sedating when first used.

5. C is correct because Dennis's increased pain indicates disease progression and the need for opioid dosages high enough to effectively control pain. Responses A and B are incorrect because Dennis's pain can likely be controlled without resorting to such invasive measures, D is incorrect because Dennis's weakness and confusion

will interfere with his ability to operate a PCA pump, and E is incorrect because attempts should be made to alleviate the distressing symptom of confusion.

6. B or C are correct because either haloperidol and midazolam *or* chlorpromazine are likely to relieve Dennis's agitation, and admission to a hospice inpatient unit may be the most appropriate setting for controlling severe agitation and relieving family stress. A is incorrect because increasing the infusion dose of hydromorphone is unlikely to reduce Dennis's agitation, D is incorrect because it is likely to result in high levels of pain, and E is incorrect because other less drastic and final solutions are likely to control Dennis's symptoms and are less likely to contribute to possible complicated grief reactions for the bereaved.

Pretest Correct Answers

1. B	16. C
2. B	17. B
3. A	18. A
4. D	19. D
5. D	20. D
6. B	21. D
7. A	22. A
8. C	23. D
9. D	24. A
10. B	25. C
11. B	26. D
12. D	27. C
13. A	28. D
14. D	29. B
15. D	30. C

Posttest

Read each item and circle the **one** correct response on the detachable answer sheet.

1. **Pain described as "shooting" or "stabbing" often results from damage to:**

   A. Bones

   B. Nerves

   C. Brain

   D. Viscera

2. **When patients are unable to swallow opioids, which of the following is an effective treatment:**

   A. Transdermal morphine

   B. Subcutaneous hydromorphone

   C. Nebulized methadone

   D. Rectal propoxyphene

3. **Which of the following classes of drugs can be effective adjuvants to morphine when treating specific types of pain?**

   A. NSAIDs

   B. Antidepressants

   C. Anticholinergics

   D. All of the above

4. **When titrating morphine, the most appropriate booster or increment dose for a patient receiving a baseline dose of 30 mg every 4 hours is:**

   A. 2 to 5 mg

   B. 10 to 15 mg

   C. 20 to 39 mg

   D. None of the above

5. **Most terminally ill patients on opioid therapy require individually titrated doses of potent bowel stimulants such as:**

   A. Senna

   B. Sorbitol

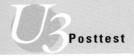

C. Psyllium

D. Docusate (Colace)

6. **An effective dose of immediate-release oral morphine provides pain relief for about:**

A. 2 hours

B. 3 hours

C. 4 hours

D. 6 hours

7. **Effective pain management depends on a comprehensive assessment of the causes of:**

A. Noncancer-related pain

B. Cancer-related pain

C. Nonphysical pain

D. All of the above

8. **Types of pain that can contribute to a patient's experience of total pain include:**

A. Physical pain

B. Social pain

C. Spiritual pain

D. All of the above

9. **When pain related to nerve damage or dysesthesia occurs, which of the following may be an effective adjuvant to morphine?**

A. Nortriptyline (Pamelor, Aventyl)

B. Scopolamine

C. Ranitidine (Zantac)

D. Naproxen

10. **To calculate an effective initial daily dose of subcutaneous hydromorphone (Dilaudid), divide the patient's daily dose of oral morphine by:**

A. 20

B. 3

C. 5

D. 2

11. **Patients treated with opioids should receive routine prophylaxis for which side effect:**

    A. Constipation

    B. Sedation

    C. Itching

    D. Myoclonus

12. **The WHO ladder of oral opioids and adjuvants has been shown to provide relief in what percent of cancer patients:**

    A. 99%

    B. 90%

    C. 75%

    D. 50%

13. **In the palliative care setting, analgesics of choice include which of the following:**

    A. Hydromorphone

    B. Meperidine

    C. Pentazocine

    D. Propoxyphene

14. **Anticholinergic drugs help with which of the following pain syndromes:**

    A. Bony

    B. Neuropathic

    C. Visceral

    D. Central

15. **When titrating morphine, the 24-hour dose can never be raised by more than:**

    A. 10%

    B. 25%

    C. 50%

    D. None of the above

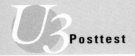

16. **A patient is receiving 60 mg of oral morphine per day. The equivalent daily dose of parenteral hydromorphone (Dilaudid) is:**

    A. 30 mg

    B. 20 mg

    C. 5 mg

    D. 3 mg

17. **The use of morphine or other opioids appropriate for treating moderate to severe pain should be saved for the last few weeks or days of the patient's life due to the risk of:**

    A. Addiction

    B. Tolerance

    C. Respiratory depression

    D. None of the above

18. **When the common side effect of constipation occurs as a result of opioid therapy, an appropriate first step is:**

    A. Digital disimpaction

    B. Soapsuds enema

    C. Trial of docusate

    D. Inquire about previous laxative use

19. **When a home hospice patient can no longer swallow, which of the following is a preferred alternative route of opioid administration:**

    A. Sublingual

    B. Intravenous

    C. Intramuscular

    D. Epidural

20. **When treating pain caused by raised intracranial pressure, an effective adjuvant to morphine would be:**

    A. Strontium 89

    B. Acetaminophen

    C. Dexamethasone

    D. Hydromorphone

21. **Which of the following most commonly occurs with opioid therapy?**

    A. Myclonus

    B. Delerium

    C. Urinary incontinence

    D. Drowsiness

22. **One oxycodone 5 mg and acetaminophen 325 mg tablet are roughly equivalent to:**

    A. 3 mg of oral morphine

    B. 7.5 mg of oral morphine

    C. 15 mg of oral morphine

    D. 4 mg of oral hydromorphone

23. **Visceral spasm pain can be effectively treated with:**

    A. An opioid plus sorbital

    B. An opioid plus metoclopramide

    C. An opioid plus oxybutynin

    D. Metoclopramide alone

24. **Neuropathic cancer pain is usually responsive to which of the following:**

    A. Morphine alone

    B. NSAIDs

    C. NSAIDs and morphine

    D. Antidepressant and morphine

25. **Opioids prescribed for pain frequently cause clinically significant:**

    A. Addiction

    B. Respiratory depression

    C. Itching

    D. Constipation

26. **In relation to oral morphine, injectable morphine is about:**

    A. Equally potent

    B. Ten times as potent

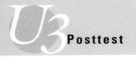

    C. Five times as potent

    D. Three times as potent

27. **Methadone should be used for relieving cancer pain when the patient has not obtained relief from:**

    A. Codeine or hydrocodone

    B. Very high dose IV/SC morphine

    C. Multidrug spinal infusions

    D. Rhizotomy or singulotomy

28. **Patients often describe bone pain as:**

    A. Shooting

    B. Deep and aching

    C. Spasms or cramping

    D. Colicky

29. **When bone pain occurs, which of the following may be an effective adjuvant to morphine?**

    A. Ibuprofen

    B. Naproxen

    C. Valdesoxib (Bexton)

    D. All of the above

30. **To calculate the equivalent parenteral dose of 30 mg of oral morphine, divide the oral dose of morphine by:**

    A. 1.5

    B. 2.0

    C. 3

    D. 6

References

[1]Jacox A, Carr DB, Payne R, et al. *Management of Cancer Pain. Clinical Practice Guideline No. 9.* AHCPR Publication N. 94-0592. Rockville, Md. Agency for Health Care Policy and Research, U.S. Department of Health and Human Services, Public Health Service; March 1994:8.

[2]Twycross R. Evaluation. In: Twycross R. *Pain Relief in Advanced Cancer.* New York: Churchill Livingston; 1994:111–128.

[3]Anand A, Carmosino L. Glatt, AE. Evaluation of recalcitrant pain in HIV-infected hospitalized patients. *J Acquired Imm D Synd.* 1994;7:52–56.

[4]Foley KM. Pain assessment and cancer pain syndromes. In Doyle D, Hanks GW, MacDonald N, eds. *Oxford Textbook of Palliative Medicine.* Oxford Medical Publications. New York. 1993:148–165.

[5]Bieri D, Reeve RA, Champion GD, et al. The Faces Pain Scale for the self-assessment of the severity of pain experienced by children: development, initial validation, and preliminary investigation for ratio scale properties. *Pain.* 1990;41:139–150.

[6]Beyer JE, Wells N. Assessment of cancer pain in children. In: Patt RB, ed. *Cancer Pain.* Philadelphia: Lippincott; 1993:57–84.

[7]Foley KM. Management of cancer pain. In DeVita VT, Hellman S, Rosenberg SA, eds. *Cancer: Principles and Practice of Oncology.* 4th ed. Philadelphia: Lippincott, 1993.

[8]Twycross R. Misunderstandings about morphine. In: Twycross R. *Pain Relief in Advanced Cancer.* New York: Churchill Livingston; 1994:333–347.

[9]Bruera E, MacMillan K, Pither J, MacDonald RN. Effects of morphine on the dyspnea of terminal cancer patients. *J Pain Symptom Manage.* 1990;5:341–344.

[10]Bruera E, MacEachern T, Ripamonti C, Hanson J. Subcutaneous morphine for dyspnea in cancer patients. *Ann Intern Med.* 1993;119:906–907.

[11]Light RW, Muro JR, Sato RI, Stansbury DW, Fischer CE, Brown SE. Effects of oral morphine on breathlessness and exercise tolerance in patients with chronic obstructive pulmonary disease. *Am Rev Respir Dis.* 1989;139:126–133.

[12]Porter J, Jick H., Boston Collaborative Drug Surveillance Program. Addiction rare in patients treated with narcotics. *N Engl J Med.* 1980;302(2):123.

[13]Definitions Related to the Use of Opioids for the Treatment of Pain: A consensus document from the American Academy of Pain Medicine, the American Pain Society, and the American Society of Addiction Medicine. 2002. www.ampainsoc.org/advocacy/opioids2.htm.

[14]*WHO Ladder: Cancer Pain Relief and Palliative Care. Technical Report Series 804.* Geneva: World Health Organization; 1990.

[15]Robb V. Working on the edge: palliative care for substance users with AIDS. *J Palliat Care.* 1995;11(2): 50–53.

[16]Gonzales GR, Coyle N. Treatment of cancer pain in a former opioid abuser: fears of the patient and staff and their influence on care. *J Pain Symptom Manage.* 1992;7(4):246–249.

[17]Lederle FA, Busch DL, Mattox KM, West MJ, Aske DM. Cost-effective treatment of constipation in the elderly: a randomized double-blind comparison of sorbitol and lactulose. *Am J Med.* 1990;89:597–601.

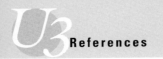
[18]Kubisty CA, Arns PA, Wedlund PJ, Branch RA. Pharmacotherapy in liver failure. Chernow B, ed. In: *Crit Care Pharmacotherapy*. Baltimore, Md: Williams and Wilkins; 1995:91–431.

[19]Rodighiero V. Effects of liver disease on pharmacokinetics: an update. *Clin Pharmacokinetics*. 1999:37(5): 399–431.

[20]Bennett WM, Aronoff GR, Morrison G, Golper TA, Pulliiam J, Wolfson M, Singer I. Drug prescribing in renal failure: dosing guidelines for adults. *Amer J Kidney Dis*. 1983;3(3):155–176.

[21]Chernow B, ed. Pharmacotherapy in renal failure. In: *Critical Care Pharmacotherapy*. Williams and Wilkins: Baltimore, Md; 1995:45–90.

[22]Swan SK, Bennett WM. Use of drugs in patients with renal failure. In: Schrier RW, Gottschalk CW, eds. *Diseases of the Kidney*, 6th ed., Vol III. Little Brown and Company: Boston; 1997:2963–3017.

[23]Pereira, J. Management of bone pain. In: Portenoy RK, Bruera E, eds. *Topics in Palliative Care* Vol 3. New York: Oxford University Press; 1998:79–116.

[24]Helweg-Larsen S, Sorensen PS. Symptoms & signs in metastatic spinal cord compression: a study of progression from first symptom until diagnosis in 53 patients. *Eur J Cancer*. 1994;30:396–398.

[25]Zeppetella G. Nebulized and intranasal fentanyl in the management of cancer—related breakthrough pain. *Palliat Med*. 2000;14:57–58.

[26]Elliott K, Foley KM. Neurologic pain syndromes in patients with cancer. In: Portenoy RK, ed. *Neurologic Clinics: Pain, Mechanisms and Syndromes*. Philadelphia: WB Saunders; 1989:333–360.

[27]Hewitt DJ, Portenoy RK. Adjuvant drugs for neuropathic cancer pain. In: Bruera E, Portenoy RK, eds. *Topics in Palliative Care—Vol. 2*. New York: Oxford University Press; 1998:31–62.

[28]Portenoy RK. Adjuvant analgesics in pain management. In: Doyle D, Hanks GW, MacDonald N, eds. *Oxford Textbook of Palliative Medicine*. New York: Oxford University Press: 1993:187–203.

[29]Storey P, Trumble M. Rectal doxepin and carbamazepine therapy in patients with cancer. *N Engl J Med*. 1992;327:1318–1319.

[30]Cassel EJ. The nature of suffering and the goals of medicine. *N Engl J Med*. 1982;306(11):639–645.

[31]Cassell EJ. Diagnosing suffering: a perspective. *Ann Intern Med*. 1999;131:531–534.

[32]Cassell EJ. *The Nature of Suffering and the Goals of Medicine*. New York; Oxford University Press: 1991; 131:531–534.

[33]Billings JA. Palliative medicine update: depression. *J Palliat Care*. 1995;11(1):48–54.

[34]Quill TE, Byock IR, ACP-ASIM End-Of-Life Care Consensus Panel. Responding to intractable terminal suffering: the role of terminal sedation and voluntary refusal of food and fluids. *Ann Intern Med*. 2000; 132:408–414.

[35]Sheard T, Maguire P. The effect of psychological interventions on anxiety and depression in cancer patients: results of two meta analyses. *Br J Cancer*. 1999;80(11):1770–1780.

[36]Ripamonti C, Zecca E, Bruera E. An update on the clinical use of methadone. *Pain*. 1997,70:109–115.

[37]Mathew P, Storey P. Subcutaneous methadone in terminally ill patients: manageable local toxicity. *J Pain Symptom Manage*. 1999;18:49–52.

[38]Bruera E., Neumann CM. Role of methadone in the management of pain in cancer patients. *Oncology*. 1999;13(9):1275–1282.

[39]Wilkinson TJ, Robinson BA, Begg EJ, Duffull SB, Ravenscroft PJ, Schneider JJ. Pharmacokinetics and efficacy of rectal versus oral sustained release morphine in cancer patients. *Cancer Chemother Pharmacol.* 1992;31:251–254.

[40]Gordon DB, Stevenson KK, Griffie J, Muchka S, Rapp C, Ford-Roberts K. Opioid equianalgesic calculations. *J Palliat Med.* 1999;2(2):209–218.

[41]Storey P, Hill HH, St. Louis RH, Tarver EE. Subcutaneous infusions for control of cancer symptoms. *J Pain Symptom Manage.* 1990;5:33–41.

[42]Twillman RK, Long TD, Cathers TA, Meuller DW. Treatment of painful skin ulcers with topical opioids. *J Pain Symptom Manage.* 1997;13:233–237.

[43]Farrar JT, Cleary J, Rauck, R, Busch M, Nordbrock E. Oral transmucosal fentanyl citrate: randomized, double-blinded, placebo-controlled trial for treatment of breakthrough pain in cancer patients. *J Natl Cancer Inst.* 1998;90(8):611–616.

[44]Streisand JB, Busch MA, Egan TD, Smith BG, Gay M, Pace NL. Dose proportionality and pharmacokinetics of oral transmucosal fentanyl citrate. *Anesthesiology.* 1998;88(2):305–309.

[45]Christie JM, Simmonds M, Patt R, Coluzzi P, Busch MA, Nordbrock E, Portenoy RK. Dose-titration, multicenter study of oral transmucosal fentanyl citrate for the treatment of breakthrough pain in cancer patients using transdermal fentanyl for persistent pain. *J Clin Oncol.* 1998;16(10):3238–3245.

[46]Raj PP. Local anesthetic blockade. In: Patt RB, ed. *Cancer Pain.* Philadelphia: Lippincott; 1993:329–341.

[47]Devulder J, Ghys L. Dhondt W, Rolly G. Spinal analgesia in terminal care: risk versus benefit. *J Pain Symptom Manage.* 1994;9(2):75–81.

[48]Fine PG. Low-dose ketamine in management of opioid nonresponsive terminal cancer pain. *J Pain Symptom Manage.* 1999;17:296–300.

[49]Cherny NI, Portenoy RK. Sedation in the management of refractory symptoms: guidelines for evaluation and treatment. *J Palliat Care.* 1994;10(2):31–38.

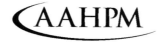

American Academy of Hospice and Palliative Medicine

UNIPAC Three: Assessment and Treatment of Pain in the Terminally Ill

Physicians are eligible to receive 6 credit hours in Category 1 of the AMA/PRA by completing and returning this posttest answer sheet to the AAHPM. The Academy will keep a record of AMA/PRA Category 1 credit hours and the record will be provided on request; however, physicians are responsible for reporting their own Category 1 CME credits when applying for the AMA/PRA or for other certificates or credentials.

Name

Street

City/State/Zip Code

Telephone

Social Security Number

Please mail this answer sheet and a check for $45.00 made out to the American Academy of Hospice and Palliative Medicine to:

**Physician Training Programs
American Academy of Hospice
 and Palliative Medicine
4700 W. Lake Avenue
Glenview, Illinois 60023-1485**

Please circle the one correct answer for each question

1. A B C D	11. A B C D	21. A B C D
2. A B C D	12. A B C D	22. A B C D
3. A B C D	13. A B C D	23. A B C D
4. A B C D	14. A B C D	24. A B C D
5. A B C D	15. A B C D	25. A B C D
6. A B C D	16. A B C D	26. A B C D
7. A B C D	17. A B C D	27. A B C D
8. A B C D	18. A B C D	28. A B C D
9. A B C D	19. A B C D	29. A B C D
10. A B C D	20. A B C D	30. A B C D